Intermittent Fasting 101 + meal plan

Contents

Introduction

Fasting has been around for millennia. It has played important roles in religious and medical literature for nearly as long. In many modern religions, fasting is the way to create spiritual connection, to find guidance or to improve mindfulness. Fasts that automatically come to mind are Lent in Catholisim and Orthodox Christianity, Ramadan in Islam or meditation fasts is some Buddhist schools. Lent lasts 40 days, and while some churches may allow more freedom with the fast, traditionally Lent required a fast where only one meal a day was eaten. During Ramadan, a month long fast, Muslims don't eat while the sun is up and then eat once the sun is down. Essentially, it is an eight to 12 hour fast, with some time to eat at night and early in the morning. In some Buddhist schools, fasting takes place to aid in meditation and spiritual practices. This often happens everyday, with the dinner meal skipped. So within religions and spiritual practices, there are many different kinds of fasts.

People have also fasted for political reasons. Perhaps most famously is Gandhi and his social protests. He fasted multiple times to protest a variety of social issues in India. There have been other hunger-strikes throughout history, where people fasted to create political change including suffragette fasting in Europe and the U.S. Many political fasts promote a feeling of guilt in those watching, and can result in change, though it has often resulted in death as well.

Medically, fasting has been around since the time of Hippocrates. Fasting was prescribed during times when the patient was sick enough that eating was considered detrimental. Past physicians believed that fasting would help with the healing of injuries and diseases. While it's unclear whether this was actually true, today, modern fasting is associated with better health improvements. In fact, intermittent fasting is our modern take on fasting for healing.

Intermittent fasting is when you choose not to eat for a specific amount of time. For example, you might fast during the evening and night hours, or you might fast every other day. In general, intermittent fasting doesn't go beyond a day of fasting. So you won't see many intermittent fasts that are 30 hours of fasting or longer. Despite how it may sound, intermittent fasting is not starvation and in fact, it's quite healthy. Intermittent fasts are about improving your health. In general, it can benefit people who are looking to lose weight, improve their blood sugar levels, and reduce their insulin resistance.

In this book, we'll cover the basics of intermittent fasting. We'll explore the different kinds, from the everyday ease of the 14/10 method to the difficult but rewarding alternate-day fast. We'll also discuss who is a perfect candidate for trying intermittent fasting, and who should refrain from it. We'll go over the benefits and risks, and explore associated research studies that demonstrate the effectiveness of intermittent fasting. Finally, we'll go into detail about schedules and possible menus for starting intermittent fasting. With this book, you'll get a thorough introduction to intermittent fasting and you'll begin your journey to starting your own intermittent fast. Let's begin.

Chapter 1: Basics of Intermittent Fasting

The beauty of social media is that ideas can be shared around the world and gain popularity very quickly. It's probably why you're here, reading this book. On social media you can find many influencers and celebrities who have tried intermittent fasting, and wholeheartedly advocate for it. Whether you want to look like the actors who play superheroes or whether you just want to get healthier, intermittent fasting can help you achieve your goals.

In the introduction, we covered how fasting was used throughout history for health, political, religious reasons. Some of these fasts are very similar to intermittent fasting. In general, intermittent fasting is when you time your eating to fit within a specific window during your day or week. Your fasting hours might just be during the night, or they might extend to a full 24 hours. When comparing intermittent fasting to religious fasting, you will see some similarities with Ramadan and Lent. During Ramadan, most people don't eat during the day, and instead eat all their meals at night. This is very similar to a 16/8 fast or even a 20/4 fast, where eating takes place in a small eight or four hour window at night. Depending on the style of Lent a person follows, you may only have one large meal in the day instead of many meals. Or you may only eat for some portion of the week and fast completely on other days. This can also be quite like intermittent fasting schedules. The difference between religious fasts and intermittent fasting are, of course, the purpose but also the timing. Religious fasts often take place for a short period of time like 20-40 days, but intermittent fasting can be a whole lifestyle change, and result in you fasting for years! It's not necessary to do it for the long term, but many people continue it even when they meet their goals for fasting.

There are so many different varieties of intermittent fasting that you'll have and easy way of finding one that fits into your lifestyle. In general, there are the methods that require you to eat in a small window everyday. These are the methods like the 12/12, 14/10, 16/8, and

20/4. In these methods, the first number is how many hours you fast, and the second number is how many hours are in your eating window. You would eat all your meals during that window of time, and during the fasting point, you would just drink liquids. The other types of fasts are those that include 24 hours of fasting between eating days. Some of these do calorie restricted meals during the fasting period so that hunger doesn't become overwhelming. Methods that do the longer 24 hour fast (with or without small meals on fasting days) include alternate day fasts, the 5:2 fast, and a general 24 hour fast. Alternate day fasts and 5:2 fasts can be similar as they take place during the course of one week. However, alternate day fasts require fasting three or four days of the week, alternating your eating days and your fasting days. While the 5:2 fast is eating normally for five days with two days of fasting spread out within the week. The 24 hour fast is one you might do once a week or even just once a month! Whichever fast you choose to do, you'll want to choose one that fits your daily life. We'll discuss these kinds of fasts later in the book.

It's important to mention that intermittent fasting isn't a diet. While people use it to receive health benefits (like they do for dieting), intermittent fasting isn't a diet at all. Most diets are focused on *what* you eat, however, intermittent fasting is all about *when* you eat. It focuses on the timing of eating to change your body's current state and bring it more into homeostasis. This can sound a little fantasy-like. Afterall, how can changing the times you eat help? Well, there's a lot of research out there about intermittent fasting, and depending on the type of fasting you follow, intermittent fasting can change your metabolism, insulin levels, and more. Let's explore more about why intermittent fasting works.

Why it Works

I can tell you that you'll lose weight on intermittent fasting and you'll become healthier. But none of that explains why? Why does fasting have such positive reviews and a following? Intermittent fasting works for so many reasons, but the main ones are the fact that it can fit in your daily life, changes some of your physiology, and can result in some caloric restriction.

Fits your life

Diets can cause a lot of changes your life. They often require specific foods that must be eaten. This can be frustrating if you live in an area where some foods aren't available. It can also be frustrating cost wise, as a lot of diet foods can be quite expensive. All of these can impact your motivation to continue dieting. Intermittent fasting doesn't cause this change to your life. You don't have to eat specific types of food when fasting. Nor do you have to spend a fortune following the schedule. All it requires of you is to eat at a specific time of day, and eat healthy meals during your eating window. This can ease the strain of starting a new fasting schedule. This also means that you won't have to do a huge change to your lifestyle.

Cravings can be a nightmare when following other styles

of dieting. You can follow a low calorie diet, but you'll probably miss eating that burger from your favorite shop, or having a scoop of ice cream with your kids. You could follow a very low or no carb diet, but you might end up missing bread, and feel a lot of restrictions when it comes to choosing your food. This can reduce the sustainability of dieting in your life. Intermittent fasting can be more reliable because you're not going to have any cravings. It doesn't restrict what you eat, which is honestly the hardest part of most conventional diets. By not restricting what you eat, you're not likely to struggle with cravings. Depending on which fasting method you choose, you might struggle with hunger, but probably not cravings.

Many of us don't follow a set eating schedule. We will often find ourselves skipping meals when we get into the flow of work or when we oversleep. Because we don't have set times to eat normally, it's really easy to change our schedule at the drop of a hat. That's why some intermittent fasts can fit into your daily schedule. If you only have to shift your eating a bit during the day, you will not struggle with the change so much. For example, if you choose to follow the 14/10 fasting schedule, you'll only have to shift your breakfast and dinner times by a couple of hours. That's so easy! Other methods of fasting can be easier, or harder depending on your current lifestyle.

Intermittent fasting doesn't require a huge shift in how you eat, unlike some other diets, which is why it can be easier to follow and fit your lifestyle better than conventional (or unconventional) diets.

Caloric restriction

Another reason that fasting works is because it can result in some unplanned calorie restriction. Calorie restriction is one of the reasons people lose weight in a regular low calorie diet. Unplanned calorie restriction means that you have a slightly lower number of daily or weekly calories than you normally eat during the day or week. Normally, an adult who is of average height and weight, eats between 2000-2200 calories a day. When fasting, you might have difficulty eating as much as you normally do during the day. Afterall, you only have a small eating window in some fasting methods. So you may end up eating 1800 calories a day. This is a significant reduction in calories, and it's all unplanned. By having this reduction, you're guaranteed to lose some weight while fasting.

In some methods of fasting, you might have some planned caloric restriction. The 24 hour methods which result in 24 hours without food, obviously result in significant weekly calorie reductions. If a healthy adult of average height and weight eats 14,000 - 15,400 calories per week, then by having some 24 hour fasts can reduce that by 2,000-6,000 calories, depending on the type of fast you choose. Alternate day fasting will provide you with way more calorie reductions than other fasts. Again, all of this reduction will result in weight loss. Because some fasts can be easier than following a consistent calorie reduction diet, fasting for this purpose can give you some good results without causing a lot of pain.

Changes your physiology

This one is a little complicated and will be discussed extensively in the chapter on benefits and risks. However, to give you a basic overview, intermittent fasting works because it can change some of your physiology and put your body back to homeostasis. By shifting your eating times, you force your body to change the way it uses its stores of glucose. This results in your body shifting from burning glucose as fuel to burning fat because the glucose stores have been used up during the fasting window. This leads to a whole host of health benefits. The best part is that these health benefits continue even after you're back to eating during your eating window. Fasting can also change your hormone levels, which also help your health and can provide so many benefits, especially to those who are already struggling with health issues. We'll cover all of this more in the chapter on benefits and risks.

Fasting is for...Everyone?

Intermittent fasting can sound rather fantastic and easy. But don't let its simple description fool you. It's a process and it can be difficult to stick with. Because of this, it's important to consider fasting carefully before you try it. Despite how much I wish I could say that fasting is for everyone, this simply isn't true. Fasting works for some, and for others it can be a dangerous affair. Here are some people who should and who should not try intermittent fasting. As always, please follow your doctor's recommendation about intermittent fasting before starting.

Let's say you already live a pretty healthy life. You exercise regularly, eat healthy meals, and are generally untroubled by any illnesses, mental or physical. If this describes you, then you could go ahead and try your fasting method of choice. You probably wouldn't have many or any side effects because you already know the basics of doing the best for your body. However, if you're like the rest of us, who have lived off fast food for most of our lives and are looking for a change, you should consider your general health and discipline towards a fast before starting. Whatever your current health status is, there are some things you should consider before starting a fast.

Consider your social priorities before you start fasting. Many people enjoy meals with their friends and family on the weekends. We also tend to eat meals with our children in the evenings. So, once you've chosen a method you're interested in, you'll need to consider how you are going to schedule your meals to fit your social engagements. If you're doing a daily fast with a method like 14/10 or 20/4, think about when you'll end your fast. Also consider if your family will be following your pattern, or if you'll be going it alone. If you're the one cooking for your family, will you be able to handle any cravings that come from watching them eat while you don't? Essentially, just consider the impact on your day to day eating habits. This will help you narrow down types of fasting that will work for you.

Beyond the social considerations, you'll have to consider your support system. It's really empowering to have people cheering for you when you're doing something hard, or new. Think about going to college and having a support system. It's so much easier than going alone. Fasting can be very difficult, and while you can go it alone, it's easier with a support system in place. This is especially true if you're planning on this being a lifestyle change. So, go through your phone contacts, and pick a few people who are reliable and can offer you support and encouragement while you start your fast. These are the people who won't make you feel guilty about not eating when they eat. They're the people who will encourage you when all you want to do is eat cake at midnight during your fasting hours. They're the people who may even choose to fast with you! Just have a support system. Furthermore, if you don't have a support system in your daily life, create your own support system by becoming active in online support groups and health coaching groups.

This is a more practical consideration but think about how your emotions might change as you fast. The first change in your eating schedule can lead to some changed moods. You might even have a change in your sleeping habits. These changes, though different, are related and can affect your life. You might be tired at work and being tired makes you feel very hungry. You may have feelings of anger when you're hungry (commonly known as being 'hangry'). You may have other shifts in your mood, but it's different for everyone. You'll need to make plans for adapting to your body's changes before starting your fast. This will help your adjustment period.

One final consideration is for anyone who does a lot of exercise or workouts. You can exercise while on your fast, but you'll need to be slow and careful when transitioning into your fast. You'll probably have to change how much protein and fiber you eat. You'll also need to plan your exercising window to coincide with your eating window. You don't want to exercise and then fast for 10 hours. Instead, you want to make sure that you have a meal after you exercise so that your body can recover. If you're an athlete, you're going to want to talk with your doctor to see if intermittent fasting will be beneficial for you before starting.

While it's important to take all of these things into consideration, fasting still isn't helpful for everyone. Here are people who shouldn't be fasting:

- Those who are pregnant or want to be pregnant.

- Those who have experienced eating disorders, anxiety, or depression (not without a doctor's recommendation).

- Those who have some medical illnesses (again, not without a doctor's recommendation).

- Those who are children. Seriously. Anyone under the age of 18 probably shouldn't fast.

Let's look at these demographics in detail to explain why fasting won't work for people in them.

Pregnancy is possibly one of the only times in your life when you can eat whatever you want, and people won't stop you. That might not be healthy though, so it's easy to see how you may want to lose weight while pregnant.

But fasting is not the way to go. Being pregnant means that you are providing the necessary nutrition for both you and your baby. Your baby's development depends entirely on what you put in your body. Fasting will result in you not intaking the right amount of food for both of you. This can negatively affect your child's development. Just like how drinking alcohol or smoking while pregnant can result in detrimental fetal development, so too can fasting. If your heart is set on trying intermittent fasting, then please try it after your baby has been weaned and you're both healthy.

If you're trying to get pregnant, then don't do intermittent fasting. There has been a couple animal studies with intermittent fasting that resulted in females having changed menstruation, low fertility, and skipped periods. While this research hasn't been carried over to humans, you don't really want to take the risk. So, wait to start intermittent fasting until another time in your life.

Intermittent fasting can mess around with your

hormones. It will shift your mood at the beginning. This can be dangerous for those who already struggle with mental illnesses or past mental illnesses. Fasting can push you into a relapse of anxiety or depression because of the change in your hormone levels. If you've experienced anxiety or depression before, you should talk to your doctor before trying fasting. You should also set up checks with your support system so they can identify if you're becoming more anxious or depressed while on a fast.

If you have ever had an eating disorder, you shouldn't fast at all. Eating disorders are all about having a really bad relationship with food, and even if you've recovered, fasting can push you back into disordered eating. Anorexia, bulimia, and binge eating are all different kinds of disordered eating. Doing a fast while experiencing one of these disorders, or after recovering from one, can push you back into disordered eating. It's easy to start fasting and then just keep going without enough eating windows if you've already experienced anorexia. Fasting could also cause a flare in binge eating

30

when breaking your fast because you're hungry from not eating for several hours. Both these situations are dangerous for your body and your mental state. So if you have experienced an eating disorder, fasting is not recommended at all, not even with a doctor's recommendation. Please don't endanger your mental health just to try and improve your physical health.

Intermittent fasting can have some good benefits for your body. If you are already struggling with some medical issues, you need to take a moment to step back and reassess your fasting ideas. Fasting can help with insulin resistance, so if you're pre-diabetic or even have been recently diagnosed with type 2 diabetes, intermittent fasting can help you, though your doctor should discuss it with you first. However, if you have been diagnosed with diabetes for a while, and have already experienced significant damage from it, then intermittent fasting shouldn't be pursued. The reason being that fasting changes your metabolic rate, insulin levels, and blood-sugar levels. If you're already struggling with maintaining these things, then fasting will throw you for a loop. Talk to your doctor if you're concerned about your weight, and they can give you some good advice for approaching a diet change or fast. Please don't just jump right in.

While diabetes is the primary concern when approaching fasting, if you have any medical difficulties, you should really talk to your doctor.

The final demographic of people who should not fast are children. There are a lot of reasons why children shouldn't fast. One of them is about people and their relationship to food. As children, we learn about food, how it makes us feel, and grow attachments to our eating habits. These habits can follow us into adulthood. Just think about it: What food brings you comfort? What do you eat when you're sad or angry? When did you learn that? A lot of this comes from childhood and what we learned during it. Comfort food literally comforts us, and the food item can be different for each person. So what we learn about food as children can follow us. If what children learn is to restrict eating, then they're not going to learn about good relationships with food. As they grow older, it will always be about restricting food. This can lead to another problem.

If children fast while growing, they'll learn that food should be restricted. This can create disordered eating, specifically anorexia. We've already discussed the importance of not fasting if you've experienced anorexia. But it's critical that children aren't taught restrictive eating in case they end up not eating at all. Now of course, fasting will not automatically cause anorexia. But it can be a trigger. Children have disordered eating for a lot of reasons, but it all narrows down to have an 'ideal' body type. If children think that fasting can get them there, then they may choose to go beyond fasting and into starvation. So it's critically important that children don't fast.

To wrap up this chapter, I urge you to first talk to your doctor before fasting. This recommendation is for anyone who is unsure about how fasting will help them, or anyone who has a current health condition. Your doctor will be able to tell you definitively about whether fasting is for you or not and help ensure that you won't affect your health negatively during your fast. Fasting can benefit a lot of people, but it's not for everyone. In the next few chapters, we're going to explore more about fasting. First, we will tackle those pesky myths you've probably heard about fasting. After that, we will examine the benefits and risks of fasting, as well as the studies that support its effectiveness. Before choosing whether you want to fast or not, check out these next two chapters. They provide some awesome information that may persuade you to try fasting.

Chapter 2: Myths of Intermittent Fasting

Myths are a beautiful thing. They're presented as absolute fact, without any proof, and we're all expected to believe them. However, they often don't have any sort of basis and can easily be debunked with just a little knowledge. This strange nature of myth can create some of our greatest stories. But in our more modern era, myths can change our beliefs and influence our decisions. Think about a lot of the myths, and often straight up lies, sent out over social media and how they negatively affect people. Myths like these can change the way we do business, take care of our families, or even approach politics or religion. The most amazing thing about myths is that we all believe them. It doesn't matter how much of a skeptic you are, there is at least one myth that you believe in. As our society keeps creating more myths, there are more and more opportunities for you to believe things that are simply untrue. This chapter is all about making sure you don't believe the myths associated with intermittent fasting.

Anytime that you have a new experience or a new idea, there are always going to be people who are willing to poke holes in it or make things up about it. I could say, "Intermittent fasting is a cure all for everything! Have appendicitis? Fast! Have a headache? Fast! Getting a little heavy while pregnant? Fast! It will solve all your problems!" And you could choose to believe me. But really, without proof you wouldn't know if I've just made these statements up or not (and yes, I did make them up, please don't fast if you're pregnant). If you choose to believe many of the other myths about fasting, then you can miss out on some great opportunities with fasting. Or worse, you could hurt yourself if you believe some of the myths. So it's important to fact check before following believing and follow myths.

While intermittent fasting is a bit new, there are still a lot of myths about it. Before starting with intermittent fasting, it's important to go through the myths so that you know exactly what is fact and what is fiction about intermittent fasting. Because we want you to believe us when we say that fasting can be beneficial, we'll include the sources for this information and research studies associated with each myth.

Myth #1: Fasting is the Same as Starvation

When many people think about fasting, they think about starvation. After all, if you're not eating, then you must be starving. However, this myth isn't true. We fast every day, for about eight hours as we sleep, and yet we don't starve. You can even skip a meal on top of your sleep time, and not starve. Beyond just this basic daily fast we all do, starvation changes our body in a different way in comparison to intermittent fasting.

In the U.S. starvation is uncommon, though it's more common to have some food insecurity. If you are experiencing starvation, you'll have not eaten for a while, or eaten very low calorie meals for several days. In fact, your starvation response starts after merely three days of not eating enough calories (Berg, Tymoczko, & Strye, 2002). During this time, you will lose weight, but you will also damage your body. In this case, your body and your brain know that you're starving, and they decide to try and save you. So your brain slows down your metabolism and sends out hormones to make you very hungry. Your body starts looking for food elsewhere. Now the science behind starvation is really detailed, but suffice it to say, normally our body gets its energy from our food, which increases our blood-glucose levels, and our insulin — all of which feeds our body. However, when starving, our body runs out of its stores of glucose and starts searching for other sources of energy. In the search for protein, your body will start cannibalizing itself, eating through important cells, and muscles. It's not a quick process, because your body still needs to function to find more food. However, without food, your body will slowly lose its functionality, leading to death.

Most of us won't starve to death in the U.S. Even when eating a very low calorie diet, our body will keep pushing us to eat and with a lot of access to food, even if most is unhealthy, we're not likely to starve to death. However, we can still feel the effects of the starvation response without the right nutrition during the day. Not only will our brain keep sending out hunger warnings, but we'll also have a shift in emotions and sometimes, cognitive function. Researchers during WWII studied starvation to determine how our bodies react to it. This study is known as the Minnesota Starvation Experiment (Keys et al., 1950), and it found some interesting effects on our brains from starvation. Many of the participants experienced emotional swings, felt cognitively foggy, and had dreams about food. They became depressed, anxious, and irritable. Physically, they experienced fluctuating body temperature, felt weak, and had reduced stamina. Their heart rate also decreased. These effects were felt in a stage of semi-starvation, where they were eating, but only a little everyday and very little of what they ate was healthy. So even when having food, we can experience the effects of starvation.

Intermittent fasting is very different from starvation because you won't be without food for three days. In fact, so long as you're following a set, healthy, fasting schedule, you will only be without food for 24 hours or less. So you will not to initiate your natural starvation response. Our body is used to normal fasting, eating states. Once you eat your last meal before a fast, your body has high blood-sugar levels, and increased insulin which are all fueling your body. The body also stores the extra glucose and puts it aside for later. After the first several hours, your body starts to reduce it's insulin levels and your blood-sugar levels also drop. Your liver releases it's stores of glucose and then your body starts using fatty tissue to continue fueling itself since it's blood-sugar levels are lower. This state is known as ketosis. Your body remains in this state for a while, even when you eat again (Berg, Tymoczko, & Strye, 2002). Because you're providing your body with food, even after 24 hours without, your body doesn't shift into its starvation response. Instead, it sticks with its stage of ketosis, with reduced insulin levels and blood-sugar levels, before getting more energy from your next meal.

It's important to note that while there are differences between starvation and fasting, any fast taken for too long will result in starvation. Any diet, where you are eating less than 1000 calories a day, puts you at risk for starting your body's starvation response. However, this response won't happen immediately. So long as you are eating something during your days, you'll be ok. In most fasts, you're going to eat your regular daily calories every day. But in some fasts like the 5:2 and the Alternate Day fasting, you'll have periods of low-calorie intake. Even during these periods, you'll only be without food for 24 hours or less. So, while doing intermittent fasting, your body shouldn't have a starvation response.

Myth #2: Fasting will Make You Gain Weight

This myth is closely related to the previous myth. It's connected to the starvation response, or as many people call it, "Starvation Mode." Starvation mode is the same thing as our starvation response, but just in a more sensationalized perspective. The general myth most people have is that fasting will put you into starvation mode, which means your metabolism slows down, you'll start hoarding all the fuel your body takes in because of the slow metabolism, and thus, you'll gain weight. Let's break this down because it's a complicated myth.

We've already covered how fasting won't put you into starvation mode if it's done correctly. So we're going to explore the metabolism aspect. When you're starving, and your body/brain starts trying to save itself, it starts to lower it's metabolism. Your metabolism is what helps you maintain your body's weight and repair your cells. It's how your body processes the food you eat and turns it into the fuel used to power your every action. During starvation, your metabolism rate will reduce because you don't have enough food to keep it running at its optimal level. This is to conserve energy for your most important living functions. Because people often think that fasting is the same as starvation, they expect your metabolism to slow while fasting, resulting in you gaining weight. This is confusing because during starvation, yes, your metabolic rate decreases, but your body is using all the stores it has. This means that there isn't any extra fuel! You will not gain weight when you're starving. It's impossible. So, carrying that belief over to fasting, just doesn't work.

In most diet culture, you'll hear people talk about 'fast' metabolism and 'slow' metabolism. Having a fast metabolism is supposed to help you lose weight because you're burning more food and fuel than you're eating and storing. A slow metabolism is supposed to make you gain weight because you're not burning enough fuel and everything extra you eat gets stored. So when people think about this myth, they think that your lack of food, will reduce your metabolism, which will lead to more food storage, with less energy and stores being used. However, this isn't true with fasting. Fasting improves your metabolism and uses your stores of energy efficiently (Patterson et al., 2016). Done right, it's likely that you will lose weight when fasting, not gain weight.

While I'd like to fully debunk this myth, there is some truth to it, and it all comes down to diet. It's possible that you can gain weight when fasting, but it's not because of your metabolic rate. If you choose to eat regular meals that exceed your daily calories, then you're going to gain weight. This is the same with any diet, any fast, or any food you eat. If you exceed what your body will use, energy/food wise, then you'll gain weight. So, it is possible that you'll gain weight when fasting. But if you do, it's not because of a lower metabolic rate, and is more because of poorly planned diet. To prevent this, it's important that you eat well-balanced nutritious foods. This will help you maintain weight, or possibly lose some if it's a shift from your normal diet. You could also combine calorie restriction with fasting, and we'll discuss this in a later chapter. Basically, if you gain weight when fasting, then it's due to diet and you'll need to watch what you eat to lose or maintain your weight.

Myth #3: Fasting is not Sustainable Long-term

There are so many diets out there that are not

sustainable. What immediately comes to mind are the types of diet where you eat only one type of food, like the cabbage soup diet. These kinds of diets are not sustainable because it's easy to start craving more types of food. Your body itself will crave the nutrients it needs, while you'll get bored with that single kind of food. A lot of diets that are fad diets aren't sustainable because they often don't provide your body with the requirements it needs to function well. This results in you being hungry and craving the foods that are prohibited in those diets. Fasting isn't like fad and doesn't restrict certain types of food. So, while you might get hungry, it's unlikely you'll have any brutal cravings. This can increase the sustainability of fasting.

Also, there are so many kinds of fasting. Some of them are really easy to incorporate into your daily life, like the 14/10 fast or the 16/8 fast. With these diets, you're simply extending your fast further than your normal eight hours of sleep. Sometimes this means eating your last meal early, or your first meal late. Because these two types are simple and easy to get into, it can be easy to maintain as well. Other types of fasting can be even easier, depending on your own personality. But the reality remains that fasting can be quickly started and maintained.

Finally, a lot of people find fasting much easier to sustain than long term calorie restriction. Long-term calorie restriction is your typical, doctor approved diet. You reduce your eaten calories by a bit every day and you lose weight. However, this can be difficult to maintain because it requires you to pick and choose what you eat carefully and can restrict social eating. In a study comparing alternate day fasting and calorie restriction, the researchers found that the participants felt the fasting was easier to sustain (Alhamdan, 2016). This has been echoed in other studies and even anecdotally. Even though hunger could be an issue with alternate day fasting, that's not always the case as participants found that their hunger on fasting days was reduced after two weeks of following the fast schedule (Klemple et al., 2010). So, fasting can be easy to start, maintain, and sustain because it doesn't restrict you.

Intermittent fasting is considered a lifestyle change. I know this is mentioned in many different diets, but with fasting, it's the easiest way to change your eating habits. It can change your health and reduce your weight. By following it in the long-term, you'll maintain all those benefits. So, fasting is and can be sustainable.

Myth #4: Fasting Causes you to Binge

This myth is based slightly on reality. It comes from how we often react when we skip a meal. We all know the feeling. You've decided to work through lunch and by the time you get home, you are dramatically dying of hunger. You go to your pantry and start gorging on anything that will fill that empty void and end hunger. When we come to, we're surrounded by the remnants of what we've eaten. It can be very surprising how much has been eaten during a moment of, what feels like, desperate hunger.

The thing that can be doubly amazing is that during this

feeling of almost insatiable hunger, our bodies are sending out signals that tell us to eat, but also to stop after a certain point. Unfortunately, most of us are incapable of hearing that, "I'm full" signal from our brains when in this state. So, we overeat. By a lot. This is a typical feeling of a binge. If we get to the point where we're very hungry, we often just start eating everything available and have a hard time stopping. So yes, it's possible that you'll binge when breaking your fast with your first meal. But it doesn't have to happen, and it doesn't happen to many people. This is because people understand how their hunger works, and how to break their fast properly to prevent binging.

When breaking your fast, you want to ease into it. Depending on what type of fast you have, you may be breaking your fast after 14 hours, or after 24 hours. So it's important to slowly break your fast. Don't just start gorging on everything you see. Take a deep breath. Have some coffee or tea. Then start eating with something small. Take a short break, and then eat a little more. Listen for your "I'm full" signal from your body. Then stop eating.

A way that can also help with this feeling is to be more mindful while you eat. Mindfulness is a common term now a days, but it can be applied to eating. Mindfulness means that you make yourself become aware of the 'now' moment. What is happening right now? What are you seeing, hearing, tasting, feeling, and smelling? At this very moment where are you and how did you get there? All of this is taking a step back and focusing on this present moment. When following mindfulness, you are not just focused on one thing, but also allowing your thoughts to come and go without you evaluating them or judging yourself. But what does this have to do with eating and binging?

Mindfulness and eating can go hand in hand. Essentially, you want to look at your current present moment, but also being aware of your body's reaction as you eat. It means eating slowly, tasting each piece of food you put in your mouth, and slowly savoring it. You could focus on your five senses while you eat and say exactly what each of them is feeling. It's also about listening to your body's reaction and looking for that full signal. Being aware of our body and how we're filling up can help us ensure that we're not giving into the hunger monster.

With mindfulness in your toolkit, you can learn what the full feeling means to your body. You can learn when to slow down and to stop eating. This can take some time. We often bypass the full feeling, so don't stress yourself as it will take time for you to get used to it. It can come along much earlier than you may have felt before, but if you can remain mindful while you eat, you can reduce the likelihood of binging. Be mindful as you eat so that you're paying attention to your hunger signals. All these things can help you break your fast without binging. So, there is some truth to this myth, but it's easily managed and prevented.

Myth #5: You Can Eat Whatever You Want

With most intermittent fasting methods, you don't have to restrict your diet when you have your eating window. This isn't in all methods, just some. The myth that you can eat whatever you want comes from this unrestriction on what you're eating. Much like the myth before this one, there is some truth to this. While fasting, you still eat whatever you want, but solely in your eating window. If you want to eat fast food every single day during your eating window, then go ahead. But...it's very likely that fasting won't help you in this case. If you're eating unhealthy foods, you're likely consuming too many calories with very little nutritious value to it. This will result in you not losing weight. In fact, you might even gain weight.

If you gain weight while fasting, look at your diet. What you eat can change how the fast will affect you. You might have better insulin levels, but you may also have a worse metabolic rate, on top of weight gain. Instead of eating a pint of ice cream every day (you know you want to), try to limit yourself and eat well-balanced meals in between your pints. If you want to lose weight, make sure that your meals are very healthy. This will ensure that the fast impacts you positively.

Myth #6: You'll be Constantly Hungry

This myth is based on fear, pure and simple. We can feel insanely hungry if we just skip a meal. What if we skip 14 hours of meals! In our minds, this sounds terrifying. We think that we'll end up being hungry all the time. Well, we will probably feel some hunger, but it won't be constant. Afterall, if you're not eating for 14 hours, then yes, you're going to feel hungry. But once you eat in your eating window, you will obviously not feel hungry anymore. If you don't believe me, then look at some of the human participants in research, or really an anecdotal evidence from those who have done intermittent fasting.

In some research, when participants completed alternate day fasting, they didn't feel very hungry once they got used to the schedule (Klemple et al., 2010). Of course, this wasn't for all participants, but for many of them, their hunger was reduced. Additionally, you can look at any blog or forum about intermittent fasting, and you'll see that a lot of people talk about how their hunger pangs were reduced after fasting for a bit. Their bodies got used to the fasting schedule, and they felt less hungry during fasting periods or days. Based on this information, it's very unlikely that you'll be constantly hungry.

Chapter 3: Benefits and Risks

After spending so much time tell you what not to believe, we've now come to the chapter that will tell you the great things about intermittent fasting. There are just so many unexpected benefits of fasting, and while I'm sure you started reading this book hoping to just lose weight with fasting, you can gain so many more health benefits than just weight loss. Unfortunately, there's nothing perfect in life, and I'm sad to say that intermittent fasting isn't perfect. There are always some risks and drawbacks of fasting. We'll also cover these in this chapter.

While reading this benefits and risks, keep in mind that not everyone will react the same way. How you react to fasting isn't going to be the same as how someone else does. So, look at your health with a critical eye and consider whether the benefits will help you or whether the risks will harm you. You can also just do a trial and error fast to see how your body will react, but always do so with wisdom.

In this chapter, we'll have some of the research studies mentioned that are about intermittent fasting. It's important to mention some of the limitations of these studies. Intermittent fasting is so recent that there isn't enough research yet on the human experience while intermittent fasting. There is some research, but not a lot. More research has been done on animals that are like humans biologically, like some apes. Some less similar animals are rodents, and there are a lot of studies on fasting with rodents. Some of these will be mentioned here and some will be human studies. But all will help explain the benefits and risks.

Benefits of Intermittent Fasting

Generally intermittent fasting has way more benefits than risks. The one everyone knows about is weight loss. But there are so many other benefits too. One of the best benefits is how intermittent fasting changes your hormone levels, so that your insulin levels are lowered.

There are also some other benefits for your heart, brain, and body.

Weight loss

Weight loss it the most well-known benefit of intermittent fasting. Even this book has the word "weight loss" in the title. During intermittent fasting, it's likely that you'll lose some weight. Whether you're following the easier 14/10 method or the harder alternate day method, you're going to lose some weight. There are a couple of reasons why this is, but the biggest one is because of calorie restriction.

Calorie restriction is one of the most common methods of weight loss recommended by doctors. We've already discussed a bit of how calorie restriction works and how unplanned versus planned calorie restriction works in fasting. In simplified 14/10 fasts and ones like it, you'll have some unplanned calorie restriction which can help you with weight loss. To get the most out of calorie restriction, you would want to follow the alternate day style of fasting. This is because there's just such a massive reduction in calories on those alternate days. Alternate day fasting has been found to be equivalent to regular, doctor approved, calorie reduction in multiple studies (Alhamdan et al., 2016; Klemple et al., 2010; Anson et al., 2003). Even better yet, because calorie reduction is interspersed with full regular meals every other day, this style of fasting is easier to stick with rather than a regular calorie restricted diet.

So, you can expect some weight loss while intermittent fasting. However, this also depends on other aspects of your lifestyle. We've talked about the importance of diet before, but we haven't talked about the importance of exercising. Doing regular exercising while intermittent fasting can also increase how much weight you lose, without losing a lot of muscle mass from the fast. You don't have to exercise heavily, but if you want to, you could go for a 30-minute walk, a bike ride or a swim. All of these can help maintain your weight loss while also maintaining your muscle mass.

The last thing to mention is that once you finish your

fasting, in the case where you're not doing this for the rest of your life, you'll be less likely to regain the weight. This isn't based on a lot of research, but some people suggest that because fasting changes how you eat and your relationship with food, you don't return to your previous style of eating. Take it or leave it, but you'll still have some improvement in your weight with intermittent fasting.

Intermittent fasting can reduce insulin levels and insulin resistance. Did you know that one-third of Americans are diagnosed with pre-diabetes? That's quite a lot and is often due to our carb and sugar laden diets. So many people in the U.S. struggle with their blood sugar levels and insulin levels. Essentially, in prediabetes your blood sugar levels are consistently higher than normal, and your body tries to fix this by increasing your insulin. Insulin is what helps your body to absorb the glucose from your food to use as energy. However, when experiencing prediabetes, your cells become resistant to the insulin. This increases the cycle again, with more insulin coming into your bloodstream and more insulin resistance occurring. This can be very problematic and result in having a diagnosis of type 2 diabetes, stroke, obesity or heart disease. Intermittent fasting can help with your insulin levels and insulin resistance.

When intermittent fasting, the blood-glucose levels can be a little more controlled, insulin resistance is reduced, and insulin itself is also reduced. This is something that has been repeated in several studies. The insulin decreases because of the way the body uses the glucose from eating during the fasting period, but it also decreases because of weight loss that is also happening. In most studies, the type of fasting used to create some of the best changes in insulin levels was alternate day fasting. This makes a lot of sense, since it's also the style of fasting that results in the most weight loss.

Improved heart health is one of the benefits that needs to be better researched in humans. However, in animals intermittent fasting is very promising for improving heart health. Intermittent fasting helps improve cholesterol levels, blood pressure, and inflammation. All of which can lead to better heart health. Obviously, this is important because since there are so many things that can negatively affect heart health. So, if intermittent fasting can help reduce these things, then you'll have a lower risk of heart disease, heart attacks, and other cardiovascular problems.

There is some research that suggests intermittent fasting can help with ageing and brain health. It has to do with how your cells recuperate from cellular stress and metabolism. The research suggests that intermittent fasting can help reduce the likelihood of Alzhemiers and Parkinson's diseases (Martin et al., 2009). While this research is very promising, there hasn't been enough human research to say this. However, the promise of better brain health is something to look forward to with intermittent fasting.

Risks of Intermittent Fasting

The risks of intermittent fasting are varied. If people fast when they shouldn't (see chapter 1), then the risks of intermittent fasting can be quite severe. However, for most people intermittent fasting isn't very risky. The risks you'll run into are bingeing, malnutrition, and difficulty with maintaining the fast. We've talked about bingeing quite extensively, so we're not going to discuss it much more. Suffice it to say, bingeing while you fast risks any of the benefits from fasting you might originally have. A bigger risk is malnutrition.

Malnutrition sounds alarming, but for the most part, you can prevent this by having well-balanced meals during your eating windows. The risk of malnutrition comes especially during the kinds of fast which include very low-calorie restriction on fasting days. Fasts like this are 5:2 fasts and alternate day fasting. If you're not eating the right nutrition throughout your week, the reduction in calories plus the poor nutrition can result in some of your dietary needs not being met. This could result in more weight loss, but also more muscle loss and other issues. To prevent this risk, you can ensure that your meals are nutritious and well-balanced. Have a variety of fruits and vegetables, try different meats and seafoods, and include grains unless you're following a specific diet like the keto diet.

Associated with malnutrition is dehydration. We get a lot of our daily water intake from the food we eat. But if you're eating a reduced amount of food during your day, or no food during your day, you're going to need to drink a lot more water than you normally do. If you're not keeping track of your hydration levels, it's possible for you to drink too little. To combat this risk, ensure that you're drinking enough by keeping a hydration journal. You could also track it in an app. Set up reminders to drink water and check your urine color. Light colored urine means good hydration, so check often despite how disgusting it might be to you.

Because fasting can be difficult to start, this can be one of the risks associated with it. You're going to feel hungry during the first couple weeks of following your fasting schedule. You may even feel uncomfortable, with mood swings, different bowel movements, and sleep disruptions. All of this can lead to you struggling with starting the fasts. They can also lead you to ignore greater warning signs that you shouldn't fast. These signs include changed heart rate, feelings of weakness, and extreme fatigue. These feelings shouldn't be ignored during the start. If you feel severely uncomfortable when you start your fast, you should stop and speak with your doctor.

Chapter 4: Styles of Intermittent Fasting

Now that you've learned the basics of intermittent fasting, it's time to go into the different types. There isn't just one style of intermittent fasting. There are basic styles like fasting for a full 24 hours, but there are also other kinds that take advantage of our normal daily activities and leave us slightly less hungry. Whichever method you choose, you'll still receive some good health benefits. There are five different varieties of intermittent fasting that will be covered in this chapter: the 14/10 method, 5:2 method, 24 Hour method, Warrior Diet method, and the Alternate Day method. These five methods have been organized from easiest to hardest.

One method that won't be discussed in this chapter is the 16/8 method. It is by far one of the easiest styles of intermittent fasting to get into and to maintain in the long-term. While we won't be covering it in this book, we did write another book that goes into the 16/8 method and provides a step-by-step guide for how to follow it. If you're interested in learning more, please look at *Intermittent Fasting 16/8: The Complete Step-by-Step Guide.*

14/10 Method

The 14/10 method takes advantage of your daily schedule to add some areas of fasting. It is a type of fasting that is called Time Restricted Eating (TRE). When reading studies about intermittent fasting, you'll see this phrase used often and it is usually referring to the 16/8, 14/10, or 12/12 methods. The 14/10 method is easy to follow, and thus, is a simple way to transition into intermittent fasting. In this method, you fast for 14 hours and then eat during a 10-hour window. It may sound a little difficult, but it isn't. Considering that you'll sleep for some of your 14 hours of fasting, you won't have to fast for as long as you think.

What many people do when they follow this style, is that they extend their fast on both sides of when they go to sleep. For instance, assuming you sleep for eight hours at night, then you'll add three hours of fasting before bed, and three hours after bed. Sometimes this doesn't work for people's schedule, especially if breakfast if important to you. In cases like this, people fast for the extra 6 hours before bed and have their last meal quite early in the day.

Because there isn't a huge shift in how you eat, when you eat, this style of intermittent fasting can be quite beneficial for people. It's something that doesn't change your normal habits very much, which is appealing to many. Afterall, if something new requires a massive change, then you'll be less likely to stick with it. The convenience of the plan also means that you're not going to have a huge difference between when you normally eat and when you eat on the fast. These smaller changes mean that you're more likely to follow the fasting plan and stay motivated to complete it.

Another benefit of this style fast is that you can still make room for social eating, unlike in other plans. If you want to have dinner with your friends, then all you must do is shift your eating and fasting windows so that you can be with your friends. Since this style of fasting doesn't require a different diet, it means that you also won't have to restrict your calories while you're eating out with your friends and family. While a diet isn't a requirement, having a well-balanced meal is recommended.

5:2 Method

This method has recently become more popular. Even comedian Jimmy Kimmel follows this style of fasting, with great results. While the 14/10 method is about when you eat, the 5:2 method is about what and when you eat. This method means that you'll eat regularly for five days a week, but then have two days where you eat a drastically reduced calorie diet. While most people eat roughly 2,200 calories in a day, while you're on the 5:2 fast, you'll eat your 2,200 calories for five days, but then eat only 500-600 calories on the two fasting days.

The benefits of having the calorie restriction twice per week means that you are more likely to lose weight, even if you overeat slightly on the days when you follow your normal diet. The 5:2 diet hasn't been more heavily researched than many other kinds of intermittent fasting, but what has been researched shows some promising studies about it. While many studies are with animals as subjects, there are a few with human participants too.

In some of the studies, it is believed that the 5:2 method can reduce tumors in breast cancer and help with other physiological issues in the body. It can help improve insulin resistance and prevent cardiovascular disease. While these studies are promising, just keep in mind that many of them revolved around animals. You can find the studies in the reference page at the end of this book, if you would like to do further research.

In general, the 5:2 method can provide you with weight loss that is on par with people who reduce calories every day. However, some people find reducing calories everyday to be very restrictive. Afterall, there's only so much you can eat on a calorie restrictive diet. However, with the 5:2 method you can eat whatever you want for your eating days, and only reduce your calories on your fasting day. While you can eat whatever you want, you should still maintain a well-balanced diet. Eating only junk food won't help with your weight loss goals, if that is the reason you're choosing to fast.

While the 5:2 method can be very beneficial, some people struggle with their first few fast days. After eating 2,000 calories on day one followed by 500 calories on day two, you can feel almost uncontrollably hungry. However, many people say (anecdotally) that the hunger fades if you keep yourself distracted. Also, so long as you follow the fast for a while, you'll soon no longer feel hungry during your fast days. All of this is anecdotal of course, but it is something to consider when choosing to fast with the 5:2 method.

24 Hour

The 24-hour fast is exactly how it sounds. You simply choose to fast entirely for 24 hours. During this fast, you don't eat at all during your fasting hours, but this doesn't mean that you can't eat during the day of your fast. One-way people cope with the 24 hours of not eating is to start their fast immediately after dinner, and then stop it at the same time the next day. This way, you're still eating on both days, just with a very long time between meals. If this is confusing to you, then here's a clarification: If you finish dinner at 7pm, then that time is your fasting start time. You would continue to fast until 7pm the next day and have your first meal right after that time. This way, you're eating something still, which might help console you.

This timing can be better than if you choose to fast from the moment you wake up one morning to the moment you wake up the next morning. This is how many people first interpret the 24-hour fast, but it is incorrect. If you followed that interpretation, then you would eat dinner at 7pm, maybe have a midnight snack at 12am, fast until you wake up at 8am, and keep fasting until 8am the next day. This places you at 32-37 hours of fasting. So, if you choose to do 24 hours fasting, then really make sure you're counting the 24 hours.

This style of fasting can give you the same benefits as other kinds of intermittent fasting. It provides an overall, weekly calorie reduction, which will lead to weight loss. However, a lot of people can struggle with this kind of fast. Going without food for 24 hours is hard, and can make you feel weak and faint, with low energy levels. On the other hand, some people find it easier to handle than the 5:2 fast, because they think having even a tiny bit of food makes you start craving more. Whichever side of the fence you fall on, the 24-hour fast is still beneficial.

Besides feeling a bit hungry during your 24 hours of fasting, there is a likelihood that you'll binge more the next day because you've simply not had anything the day before. Even if you binge a bit, it's unlikely that you'll eat a full day's worth of extra calories. So, you'll still have a weekly calorie reduction.

The Warrior Diet

The Warrior Diet is labelled as a diet, but it's typically a style of intermittent fasting. The Warrior Diet is called such because it's believed to follow the eating habits of ancient warriors. It's based on the belief that warriors would eat very little during the day and then overeat at night in a 'feast.' Essentially, this leads to a 20:4 fast, with 20 hours of fasting, and four hours of eating. Having only four hours to eat can be very difficult for people, especially if you're supposed to overeat. For many of us, having a heavy meal at nighttime can interrupt our sleep habits and can make us feel ill. For others, having to eat so much after a long fast can lead to some gastric distress. So, the Warrior Diet has some areas that people may struggle with.

What you eat is just as important as when you eat during this fast. It's recommended you eat unprocessed foods, with a lot of raw vegetables and fruits. During your 20 hours of fasting, you can eat tiny amounts of fruit and vegetables, but some people will find it difficult to sustain their day on this. With the change in diet and eating time, the Warrior Diet will supposedly cause a clearer mind and better cellular repair. This is possible, since eating less processed food can result in ketosis which helps with cellular repair, and there is some research supporting intermittent fasting for improved brain function. While there isn't a lot of research on the Warrior Diet itself, because it is technically a type of intermittent fasting, some of the research found could carry over to the Warrior Diet. So, it's possible it will lead to weight loss but it's also possible that it won't. There simply isn't enough research out there to promote a 20:4 fast.

The Warrior Diet might work in theory, but it will depend on the type of person who is following it. If you have a lot of dedication, motivation, and a good understanding of nutrition, you could do very well with the Warrior Diet. However, if you're leaving a carbohydrate heavy diet, with three meals a day, the Warrior Diet can be a severe change which can reduce your motivation to continue. Beyond this, with only a four-hour eating window, it can be difficult to do social eating activities, like having brunch, or eating out with your co-workers for lunch. This can strain the motivation and sustainability of those who are trying to follow the diet. This is why it's one of the harder versions of intermittent fasting to follow.

Alternate Day

Alternate Day fasting is like an extended version of the 5:2 method. There's actually a lot of research that supports alternate day fasting, and it's considered to be really good for reducing belly fat in people who are very obese. Even if weight is maintained, there's a good chance that alternate day fasting can lead to better health overall. It can reduce insulin levels and insulin resistance and can help the brain handle cell stress (Anson et al., 2003). There are a lot of studies about it, but as mentioned before, some of these studies are animal studies. However, they provide some promising implications for how alternate day fasting can help humans.

In this fast, you are fasting every other day, and eating your regular portions on your off days. This means that you have an overall reduced calorie load during the week. This is similar to a regular calorie reduction diet, where calories are reduced everyday. So, the weekly calorie restriction can be the same in both the fast and the diet. However, people generally find alternate day fasting easier to follow than calorie restricted diets. There are some people who dislike the alternate day fast because it can be very difficult to go hungry during the fasting days. This hunger doesn't always get easier as the weeks go on. This can strain people's motivation to continue the fast. Some people combat this by eating a reduced calorie meal on fasting days. In this case, this adaptation makes the alternate day fast like the 5:2 fast, with just extra days of fasting.

Because there is a significant calorie reduction, it's important that the meals you eat are nutritious. You don't want to be undernourished while following this fast. Additionally, if you're already at a healthy weight, this fast may make you lose weight that you can't afford to lose. So be careful when approaching this fast. However, if you are very overweight, then this fast can help you. Just work with your doctor to figure out if this fast will be of benefit to you. As mentioned earlier, there is significant research associated with alternate day fasting, and a lot of it is positive. So, this style of fasting can bring you significant benefits.

To conclude this chapter, there are several different options for following an intermittent fast. You should choose the fasting method that works for you and your lifestyle. If you're a very social eater, then choose a fast like the 14:10 fast or perhaps the 5:2 fast. If you're very determined, have great discipline, and can maintain motivation, then choose a fast like the 24-hour, alternate day, or the Warrior Diet. Either way, you'll likely get some benefits from these fast choices. But with benefits, always comes risks. These fasts all have some risks associated and it's important to know them before choosing to follow intermittent fasting. In the next chapter, we'll be discussing the benefits of fasting in general, and explore the risks associated with fasting.

Chapter 5: Transitioning into Intermittent Fasting

Now we get into the fine print of intermittent fasting. You've learned all the basics of intermittent fasting in general, but it's time to learn how to start your fasts. In this chapter, we'll look at transitioning schedules for each kind of fast. Use the schedules to help you determine which fasts will work for you and which ones are not going to work for your lifestyle.

One recommendation I have for you is to track your fast by maintaining a journal. Your journal can help you with your schedule, but also can be a consistent record of which styles have worked for you, which have not, and where you are struggling with the fasts. When you have your journal set up, start by including your chosen fasting schedule and why you've chosen that one. Also add your goals to the journal and write down what works and doesn't for you. Keep it regularly updated and you'll have a beautiful record of your fasting journey.

Before looking at our schedules, there are some things to keep in mind.

- Each of the schedules below will give you some variation of how to start and transition into them. So, when you choose your schedule, you'll have plenty of options to choose from. However, if you don't find a schedule that works for you, then create your own! Each one is personal.

- The schedules don't have to be permanent. Don't feel like you're committed to one type of schedule simply because you've already been using it for several weeks. If it's not working, change it up and choose a different schedule. And if you want to eat out during your fasting window, then just shift your fasting and eating time to fit your social schedule. This isn't an inseparable marriage. Simply choose and adapt your schedule to fit you and don't feel any guilt about changing them as you go along.

- Ideally, you want to transition slowly. So, each

schedule will demonstrate a slow transition into the fast. If you don't want to go slow, that's your choice. But going slow will help you ease into the fast and reduce the likelihood of feeling those negative emotions we discussed before. Each of these schedules shows a transition period of two weeks before you're fully following the schedule.

Transitioning into 14:10

When transitioning into the 14:10 schedule, you have a variety of options. You can choose to have an early eating schedule, where your first meal is very early in the morning. You could follow the mid-day eating schedule, or you could follow the late day eating schedule. Choose the one that fits your lifestyle. If you're a shift worker, the late day eating schedule might work best for you. If you're an early morning person, then that schedule will be your best bet. So, choose the one that fits you best.

Early Eating Schedule

If you want to follow your body's natural rhythm of being more active during the early morning, then this is the schedule for you. It's also great because it gives you a decent time in the evening where you'll be without food, which can help you when you sleep. In this schedule, you'll start eating at 7am and end at 5pm. This is a slow transition, so it's a one hour transition every couple of days over the course of two weeks.

Time	Day 1-3	Day 4-6	Day 7-9	Day 10-12
7 A.M.	Wake up Eat	Wake up Eat	Wake up Eat	Wake up Eat
9 A.M.	Eat	Eat	Eat	Eat
11 A.M.	Eat	Eat	Eat	Eat

1 P.M.	Eat	Eat	Eat	Eat
3 P.M.	Snack	Eat	Eat	Eat
5 P.M.	Eat	Eat	Eat	Eat before 5
7 P.M.	Eat	Eat	Fast	Fast
9 P.M.	Eat	Fast	Fast	Fast
10 P.M.-	Sleep/ Fast	Sleep/ Fast	Sleep/ Fast	Sleep/ Fast

Once you've transitioned into the fast, here is what your week will look like:

Time	12 A.M. - 7 A.M.	7 am	12 P.M.	4 P.M.	5 P.M. - 12 A.M.

Monday - Sunday	Fast/sleep	Breakfast	Large meal	Last meal, finished by 5 P.M.	Fast/Sleep

Mid-day Eating Schedule

The mid-day eating schedule works for people who aren't morning people. It's also something that you can follow on the weekends, if you want a later start to your day. This schedule is also great because you can have more of a social life than in the early eating schedule. After all, most people eat dinner out socially usually after 5pm. Again, this schedule is a transition over the course of a couple of weeks. This may help reduce your feelings of discomfort as you transition. In this schedule, you start eating at 10am and finish your last meal by 8pm.

Time	Day 1-3	Day 4-6	Day 7-9	Day 10-12
6 A.M.	Sleep/Eat	Sleep/ Fast	Sleep/ Fast	Sleep/ Fast
8 A.M.	Eat	Eat	Fast	Fast
10 A.M.	Eat	Eat	Eat	Eat
12 P.M.	Eat	Eat	Eat	
2 P.M.	Snack	Snack		Eat
4 P.M.	Eat	Eat	Eat	Eat

6 P.M.	Eat	Eat	Eat	
8 P.M.	Eat	Eat	Eat	Eat before 8
10 P.M. -	Sleep/Fast	Sleep/Fast	Sleep/Fast	Sleep/Fast

Once you've transitioned into the fast, here is what your week will look like:

Time	12 A.M. - 7 A.M.	10 A.M.	2 P.M.	7 P.M.	8 P.M. - 12 A.M.
Monday - Sunda	Fast/sleep	Breakfast	Large meal	Last meal, finished by 8	Fast/Sleep

y				P.M.	

Evening Eating Schedule

Many people have difficulty eating late at night. However, if you're a night owl and want to have later meals, this schedule is for you. There are some things to notice about this schedule. First is that our bodies don't normally metabolize food efficiently at night. So, you may have difficulty sleeping if you eat too late, and you won't have the same benefits with glucose as you would by eating early in the day. However, this schedule is perfect if you plan on partying with your friends late at night, or if you work unconventional hours. Just like before, this fast transitions over the course of a couple weeks. Your eating window starts at 2pm and ends at 12am.

Time	Day 1-3	Day 4-6	Day 7-9	Day 10-12
12 A.M - 6 A.M.	Sleep/ Fast	Sleep/ Fast	Sleep/ Fast	Sleep/ Fast
8 A.M.	Eat	Fast	Fast	Fast
10 A.M.	Eat	Eat	Fast	Fast
12 P.M.	Eat	Eat	Eat	Fast
2 P.M.	Snack	Eat	Eat	Eat
4 P.M.	Eat	Eat	Snack	Eat
6 P.M.	Eat	Snack	Eat	Eat
8 P.M.	Eat	Eat	Eat	Eat

10 P.M.	Eat	Eat	Eat	Eat
12 A.M.	Eat	Eat	Eat	Eat before midnight

Once you've transitioned into the fast, here is what your week will look like:

Time	12 A.M. - 8 A.M.	8 A.M. - 2.P.M.	2 P.M.	7 P.M.	11 P.M. - 12 A.M.
Monday - Sunday	Fast/sleep	Fast	Breakfast	Large meal	Last meal, finished by midnigh

				t

With these three schedules, you have a variety of opportunities to fast following the 14/10 method. Make sure that you take the time to make these schedules yours. Adapt them to your schedule and your family situation. You can also shift your schedule over a couple of days. If the early morning schedule appeals to you, but you like having dinner out with friends every Friday night, then you may choose to shift your eating windows for the weekend. This way you're still fasting for 14 hours and eating within a 10-hour window.

Transitioning into 5:2

The 5:2 schedule is different from the 14/10 schedule. It doesn't require a daily fast, but instead requires two days of fasting within the week. During those two days, you'll eat just 500-600 calories for that day. In this section, we'll look at two possible schedules for your 5:2 fast. The first schedule is one where you fast on Mondays and Thursdays. The second option is a fast on Wednesdays and Saturdays. If you choose to create your own schedule, make sure that you have a couple of days between each fasting day. Don't fast for Saturday and Sunday. That's 48 hours with limited calories and isn't good for your body. You'll also feel incredibly hungry by the time you eat on Monday. So, if you are following your own schedule, make sure you have a couple of days between each fasting day.

Monday and Thursday fasting days

This schedule is perfect for those who are comfortable being at work without much food. For some of us, this doesn't work. However, if you feel very comfortable with it, then this schedule will work for you. Remember that during your fasting days, you can eat 500-600 calories. During your eating days, you can eat what you want, but try not to overeat or you'll undo the good you did during

93

your fast. This schedule will transition you over the course of a couple of weeks.

Week 1

Time	Mon	Tue	Wed	Thurs	Fri	Sat	Sun
8 A.M.	Fast	Eat all day	Eat all day	Fast	Eat all day	Eat all day	Eat all day
12 P.M.	Eat 800 calories	Eat	Eat	Eat 600 calories	Eat	Eat	Eat
4 P.M.		Eat	Eat		Eat	Eat	Eat

8 P.M.	Eat 400 calories	Eat	Eat	Eat 400 calories	Eat	Eat	Eat
10 P.M.	Sleep / Fast	Sleep/ Fast	Sleep/ Fast	Sleep / Fast	Eat	Eat	Eat
12 P.M	Sleep / Fast	Sleep/ Fast	Sleep/ Fast	Sleep / Fast	Sleep/ Fast	Sleep/ Fast	Sleep/ Fast

Week 2

Time	Mon	Tue	Wed	Thurs	Fri	Sat	Sun
8	Fast	Eat	Eat	Fast	Eat	Eat	Eat

A. M.		all day	all day		all day	all day	all day
12 P.M.	Eat 400 calories	Eat	Eat	Eat 400 calories	Eat	Eat	Eat
4 P.M.	Fast	Eat	Eat	Fast	Eat	Eat	Eat
8 P.M.	Eat 400 calories	Eat	Eat	Eat 300 calories	Eat	Eat	Eat
10 P.M.	Sleep / Fast	Sleep/ Fast	Sleep/ Fast	Sleep / Fast	Eat	Eat	Eat

12 P.M	Sleep/ Fast	Sleep/ Fast	Sleep/ Fast	Sleep/ Fast	Sleep/ Fast	Sleep/ Fast	Sleep/ Fast

You can see in this schedule; you're increasing your fasting time from week one to week two on your fasting days. There's also a mid-day fast within week two. When you fully transition into your fast, your week will look like this:

Mon	Tue	Wed	Thur	Friday	Sat	Sun
Fast day: Eat 500-600 calories	Eating day: Eat what you want, but	Eating day	Fast day: Eat 500-600 calories	Eating day: Eat what you want, but	Eating day	Eating day

throu gh the day, or eat one large meal	don't overea t. Break your fast careful ly		throu gh the day, or eat one large meal	don't overea t. Break your fast careful ly		

In the schedule above, you should have noticed the additional note to break your fast carefully. Because you'll be breaking your fast after a day with very low calories, you want to break it slowly. Start your breakfast with something that is light, not too heavy, and not something sugary. If you don't, you may feel some gastric upset and nausea. So, break your fast with some tea or bone broth, have a bit of yogurt and nuts, or something else light for you. Once you break your fast, you can eat normally throughout the day. There's more about breaking your fast in the section on transitioning into the 24 hours fast.

Wednesday and Saturday fasting days

This schedule works well for those who want to fast over a weekend day. This can be great if you tend to feel faint or very hungry when fasting. It can also be less distracting than if you're sitting at work watching everyone eat donuts and coffee while you're fasting. This schedule might not work for you if you're a very social eater over the weekends. So, take that into consideration before choosing this schedule.

Week 1

Time	Mon	Tue	Wed	Thurs	Fri	Sat	Sun
8 A. M.	Eat all day	Eat all day	Fast	Eat all day	Eat all day	Fast	Eat all day

12 P.M.	Eat	Eat	Eat 800 calories	Eat	Eat	Eat 600 calories	Eat
4 P.M.	Eat	Eat	Eat	Eat	Eat	Eat	Eat
8 P.M.	Eat	Eat	Eat 400 calories	Eat	Eat	Eat 400 calories	Eat
10 P.M.	Slee p/ Fast	Slee p/ Fast	Sleep / Fast	Slee p/ Fast	Eat		Eat
12 P.M	Slee p/	Slee p/	Sleep /	Slee p/	Slee p/	Sleep /	Slee p/

	Fast	Fast	Fast	Fast	Fast	Fast	Fast

Week 2

Time	Mon	Tue	Wed	Thurs	Fri	Sat	Sun
8 A.M.	Eat all day	Eat all day	Fast	Eat all day	Eat all day	Fast	Eat all day
12 P.M.	Eat	Eat	Eat 400 calories	Eat	Eat	Eat 400 calories	Eat
4 P.M.	Eat	Eat	Fast	Eat	Eat	Fast	Eat

8 P.M.	Eat	Eat	Eat 400 calories	Eat	Eat	Eat 300 calories	Eat
10 P.M.	Sleep/ Fast	Sleep/ Fast	Sleep/ Fast	Sleep/ Fast	Eat	Fast	Eat
12 P.M	Sleep/ Fast	Sleep/ Fast	Sleep/ Fast	Sleep/ Fast	Sleep/ Fast	Sleep/ Fast	Sleep/ Fast

When you fully transition into your fast, your week will look like this:

Mon	Tue	Wed	Thur	Friday	Sat	Sun

Eating day	Eating day	Fast day: Eat 500-600 calories through the day, or eat one large meal	Eating day: Eat what you want, but don't overeat. Break your fast carefully	Eating day	Fast day: Eat 500-600 calories through the day, or eat one large meal	Eating day: Eat what you want, but don't overeat. Break your fast carefully

In both these fasting plans, you'll notice that there are some recommendations for how many calories to eat on your fasting days as you transition. These are recommendations, with the hope that it will be easier to do the full fast in week three. However, shifting to such few calories can be a little jarring. So, if you need to take it slower, go ahead! Do whatever help your body adjust to the fast best. These plans put 'breakfast' as the largest meal and it's the one that shifts to fewer and fewer calories for the fasting days. This is because it's better to have a larger meal in the morning than in the evening.

For your fasting days, you can choose to eat your 500-600 calories all in one meal, or you may choose to break it up over a couple meals/snacks. In these plans we put them as two meals, but it can also be an all-day grazing situation. You could just snack on fruits and vegetables throughout the day, with some protein interspersed. This can help you feel fuller throughout your day, rather than just eating one large meal. However, you want to choose what you'll do based on your situation. We'll discuss some options for meals in a later chapter.

Transitioning into 24 Hour Fast

This fast is very flexible, as there's no requirement for which day you choose to fast. The only thing to keep in mind is that you don't want to fast two days in a row. Keep it at just 24 hours, and no longer. This is to ensure that you're not starting your body's starvation response with further fasting.

For this fast style, there is only one example schedule. This is just to give you an idea of how to time your 24 hours, so you still have a meal everyday, while still having a 24-hour window where you're not eating. In this schedule, the fasting days are on Saturday and Tuesday. Because there isn't a set day requirement for this fast, you could choose just to fast one day, or two days in the week. If you want to fast three days, that's moving into the alternate day fasting, which we'll talk about later in this chapter.

Here is your schedule into 24 hours fasting. There isn't a transitioning period for this one, since when you choose to fast is completely random.

Time	Mon	Tues	Wed	Thur	Fri	Sat	Sun
12 A.M -6 A.M.	Sleep / Fast	Sleep / Fast	Sleep / Fast	Sleep / Fast	Sleep / Fast	Sleep / Fast	Sleep / Fast
8 A.M.	Eat all day	Eat	Fast	Eat all day	Eat	Fast	Eat all day
10 A.M.	Eat	Finish eating by 12. P.M.	Fast	Eat	Eat	Fast	Eat

12 P.M.	Eat	Fast	Break Fast	Eat	Eat	Fast	Eat
2 P.M.	Eat	Fast	Eat	Eat	Eat	Fast	Eat
4 P.M.	Eat	Fast	Eat	Eat	Eat	Fast	Eat
6 P.M.	Eat	Fast	Eat	Eat	Finish eating by 8 P.M.	Fast	Eat
8 P.M	Eat	Fast	Eat	Eat	Fast	Break k	Eat

.						Fast	
10 P.M.	Eat	Fast	Eat	Eat	Fast	Eat	Eat

For this kind of fast, choose to fast on the days when you won't need to do a lot of physical work. If your job if physically demanding, then fast on weekends or days when you won't work. If you just like working out a lot, then on your fasting days, you'll want to take it easy or skip all together. Whatever you do, if you decide to exercise while on this fast, make sure it's right before you break your fast. You want to eat a good mix of protein and fiber after exercising to help your muscles recover.

With a 24 hour fast, it's very important that you maintain your hydration levels. Have water, tea, and black coffee during your fast. This will help with your hunger, but also help you stay hydrated. Becoming dehydrated will cause you some damage, especially because you're not getting your hydration from food. So, keep drinking liquids throughout your day, and regularly check your hydration.

In this fast and in other 24-hour style fasts, you will want to be careful with how you break your fast.

What to Eat to Break your Fast

Once you've survived your 24 hours fast, it's time to eat again. You're going to feel hungry. There's no way around it but you might feel intensely hungry. The last thing you want to do is gorge yourself on all the food. It's possible it will all just right back up if you do so, and you'll also lose some of the benefits you received from the fast in the first place. To prevent difficulty with eating again, it's important to take things slow as you break your fast.

Start by eating a little snack such as some blueberries.

Starting with a liquid like water, tea, or coffee can be a great option. Another option is to have bone broth. This will help you feel fuller, but also provide you with some good nutrients for starting your eating window. After having some liquids and a small snack, 10 minutes later eat something a bit more substantial.

You're going to want to change your food type for breaking your fast. While a bacon burger will be so tempting, it's not the best choice to break your fast. It's way too heavy, too fatty, and too much for your first meal. It can make you feel bloated, have indigestion, or make you sick to your stomach. So, if you're desperate for that burger, eat it later, long after you've broken your fast. Instead of a burger, have some light proteins and fibers. Choose some fruit that aren't going to spike your blood-sugar, like raspberries, and eat them with some yogurt. Add some sunflower or flax seeds to your yogurt for added nutrition.

Some people have a lot of difficulty with eating something sugary or full of carbs after a fast. It can cause you to feel bloated and miserable. It spikes your blood sugar very quickly after a period of having lower blood-sugar levels because of your fast. This can be jarring and result in some negative physical responses. However, some people are really used to eating sweetened cereal for breakfast or even PopTarts. If you are desperate for your oatmeal in the morning after a fast, then go ahead and eat some. Check how your body feels while and after eating. This can give you a good idea for how you respond to eating these foods after a long fast. If you find that you feel miserable, then you know to avoid those foods when breaking your fast. If you feel fine, then go ahead and stick with your normal routine.

Transitioning into the Warrior Diet

This section is more about a 20:4 intermittent fast, rather than the warrior diet itself. The warrior diet has its own transitioning recommendations, which may or may not work for everyone. It can be intense, requiring significant diet changes while also changing when you eat — all of which take place at the same time and right at the beginning of the diet. So, this can be difficult to start. For this reason, this section will talk about how to transition into a 20:4 fasting schedule over the course of a couple weeks.

Like we did for the 14:10 fast, we'll provide you with some different fasting schedules that might fit your lifestyle. Once you've transitioned, you'll have a 20-hour fasting window.

Early eating schedule

This schedule is perfect if you don't want to skip breakfast. In fact, there are a lot of people that say you shouldn't skip breakfast at all. This is partially because of your circadian rhythm. Your body is more primed to activity in the morning than in the evening. So, eating your meals in the morning can have the most benefit to you. By following the early morning schedule, you won't be going to bed on a full stomach. Sleeping with so much digestion happening can be nightmare inducing. Literally. But it can also cause you to have a restless sleep, have less energy in the morning, and just in general feel terrible. So, the early morning eating schedule is perfect for those who want to avoid these difficulties. This fasting schedule opens the eating window at 7am and ends the eating window at 11am

Here is your schedule for the 20 hours fast:

Time	Day 1-3	Day 4-6	Day 7-9	Day 10-12
7 A.M.	Wake up Eat	Wake up Eat	Wake up Eat	Wake up Eat
9 A.M.	Eat	Eat	Eat	Eat
11 A.M.	Eat	Eat	Eat	Eat before 11

1 P.M.	Eat	Eat	Eat	Fast
3 P.M.	Snack	Eat	Fast	Fast
5 P.M.	Eat	Eat	Fast	Fast
7 P.M.	Eat	Fast	Fast	Fast
9 P.M.	Fast	Fast	Fast	Fast
10 P.M.-	Sleep/ Fast	Sleep/ Fast	Sleep/ Fast	Sleep/ Fast

As you can see in this schedule, it's a very significant change every three days. This should help you shift into your 20 hours of fasting, but if you're finding it difficult, then go slower before going into the 20 hours.

Once you've transitioned into the fast, you'll have a weekly schedule that looks like this:

Time	12 A.M. - 6 A.M.	7 A.M.	10 A.M.	11 A.M.	10 P.M. -
Monday - Sunday	Fast/sleep	Breakfast	Last meal, finished by 11 A.M.	Fast	Fast/sleep

This schedule can put a strain on your social eating. If you want to eat out with friends, you can adjust your eating window, but don't do a drastic adjustment. If you abruptly change your eating window, then it's possible that you'll have more than 24 hours of fasting and this can be very jarring if you're not prepared for it.

Mid-day eating schedule

This fasting window is perfect for those who are

comfortable with eating a lot during work. It's also a good window if you want to have social lunches to eat with your friends and family. Because this window is still early in the day, you'll avoid the difficulties with late night eating mentioned in the first schedule. This fasting schedule opens your eating window at 11am and closes it at 3pm.

Here is your fasting schedule for the midday eating window:

Time	Day 1-3	Day 4-6	Day 7-9	Day 10-12
6 A.M.	Sleep/ Fast	Sleep/ Fast	Sleep/ Fast	Sleep/ Fast
9 A.M.	Eat	Eat	Fast	Fast
11 A.M.	Eat	Eat	Eat	Eat

1 P.M.	Eat	Eat	Eat	Eat
3 P.M.	Snack	Snack	Eat	Eat before 3
5 P.M.	Eat	Eat	Eat	Fast
7 P.M.	Eat	Eat	Fast	Fast
9 P.M.	Eat	Fast	Fast	Fast
10 P.M.-	Sleep/ Fast	Sleep/ Fast	Sleep/ Fast	Sleep/ Fast

Once you've transitioned into your fast, you'll have a weekly schedule that looks like this:

Time	12 A.M. - 6 A.M.	7 A.M. -11	11 A.M.	3 P.M.	10 P.M. -

		A.M.			
Monday - Sunday	Fast/sleep	Fast	Breakfast	Last meal, finished by 3 P.M.	Fast/sleep

Evening eating schedule

This schedule is perfect if you do a lot of social eating and want to be able to eat with your friends and family at nighttime. The downside to this schedule is that it ends late enough that you may experience some discomfort while you sleep. Many people have nightmares if they eat before bed, especially if they eat a lot. You may also have a very restless sleep. If you stay up all night, then this fast will work for you. In this schedule, your eating window opens at 6pm and closes at 10pm

Here is your fasting schedule for late evening meals:

Time	Day 1-3	Day 4-6	Day 7-9	Day 10-12
6 A.M.	Sleep/ Fast	Sleep/ Fast	Sleep/ Fast	Sleep/ Fast
8 A.M.	Fast	Fast	Fast	Fast
10 A.M.	Eat	Fast	Fast	Fast
12 P.M.	Eat	Eat	Fast	Fast
2 P.M.	Snack	Eat	Eat	Fast
4 P.M.	Eat	Eat	Eat	Fast

6 P.M.	Eat	Eat	Eat	Eat
8 P.M.	Eat	Eat	Eat	Eat
10 P.M.	Eat	Eat	Eat	Eat before 10 P.M.
11 P.M. -	Sleep/ Fast	Sleep/ Fast	Sleep/ Fast	Sleep/ Fast

Once you've transitioned into your fast, you'll have a weekly schedule that looks like this:

Time	12 A.M. - 6 A.M.	7 A.M.- 12 P.M.	12 P.M.- 6 P.M.	10 P.M.	10 P.M. -

Monday - Sunday	Fast/sleep	Fast	Fast	Break fast	Last meal, finished by 10 P.M.

While the warrior diet is a kind of intermittent fasting, it's very difficult to follow and not recommended for most people. You'll need to eat a lot during those four hours to maintain your nutrition, and this can be quite difficult. Eating 2,000 calories within four hours is nearly impossible, so you'll have significant calorie reductions during your day. You need to ensure you eat at minimum, 1300 calories during your eating windows to help you stay healthy. Each of your meals also must be nutritious and well-balanced. If you only eat food without a lot of nutrients, but with a lot of calories, you'll end up not having enough nutrients in your diet.

During your fasting window, the official warrior diet

recommends you have liquids like broth, juice, water, and vegetable juice. They also recommend eating some dairy during the fasting window. Dairy like hard boiled eggs is allowed during the fasting period. This might make it a bit easier to follow the rest of the schedule. It will also help ease your hunger.

If you want to try this type of fast, take your time and pay close attention to your body. Check-in with yourself regularly. If you find that people are becoming increasingly annoying and irritating to you, and that the hunger never ends, then this fast is not for you. Ease back into a simpler 14:10 fast or 16:8 fast.

Transitioning into Alternate Day Fasting

Alternate day fasting is the kind of fast that has the most research associated and can lead to the most gains with fasting. So, it's easy to see how it can be a very popular choice. Even though it's beneficial, it's also hard to follow. It is a 24-hour style of fast, but it happens every other day instead of just once or twice a week. The transition into this will be like the 24 hours fast. There isn't going to be a huge transition period. You just must dive in. You'll have a meal every day, but during your fasting window, you won't have any meals. This is the traditional way to do alternate day fasting. If this is too difficult for you, you could add 500 calories to your fasting days, like you would for the 5:2 fasting method.

Here is one possible fasting schedule with alternate day fasting:

Time	Mon	Tues	Wed	Thur	Fri	Sat	Sun	Monday
12 A. M - 6 A. M.	Sleep/ Fast	Sleep/ Fast	Sleep/ Fast	Sleep/ Fast	Sleep/ Fast	Sleep/ Fast	Sleep/ Fast	Sleep/ Fast

8 A. M.	Eat	Fast	Eat all day	Eat	Fast	Eat all day	Eat	Fast
10 A. M.	Eat	Fast	Eat	Eat	Fast	Eat	Eat	Fast
12 P. M.	Eat	Fast	Eat	Eat	Fast	Eat	Eat	Fast
2 P. M.	Eat	Fast	Eat	Eat	Fast	Eat	Eat	Fast
4 P. M.	Eat	Fast	Eat	Eat	Fast	Eat	Eat	Fast

6 P. M.	Finish eating by 8 P.M.	Fast	Eat	Finish eating by 8 P.M.	Fast	Eat	Finish eating by 8 P.M.	Fast
8 P. M.	Fast	Break Fast	Eat	Fast	Break Fast	Eat	Fast	Break Fast
10 P. M.	Fast	Eat	Eat	Fast	Eat	Eat	Fast	Eat

In this schedule, you have some days without any fasting at all, but each day also has an eating window. This can be helpful if you struggle with having no food at all during the day. You can see how the next week starts on the opposite schedule. The whole point is to alternate days for eating and fasting, so each week will be a little different.

If you want to follow a schedule that looks more like an alternate day one, then you can follow this schedule:

Time	Mon	Tues	Wed	Thur	Fri	Sat	Sun	Monday
12 A.M - 6 A.M.	Sleep/ Fast	Sleep/ Fast	Sleep/ Fast	Sleep/ Fast	Sleep/ Fast	Sleep/ Fast	Sleep/ Fast	Sleep/ Fast
8 A.M.	Eat all day	Fast all day	Eat all day	Fast all day	Eat all day	Fast all day	Eat all day	Fast all day

10 A. M.	Eat	Fast	Eat	Fast	Eat	Fast	Eat	Fast
12 P. M.	Eat	Fast	Eat	Fast	Eat	Fast	Eat	Fast
2 P. M.	Eat	Fast	Eat	Fast	Eat	Fast	Eat	Fast
4 P. M.	Eat	Fast	Eat	Fast	Eat	Fast	Eat	Fast
6 P. M.	Eat	Fast	Eat	Fast	Eat	Fast	Eat	Fast

8 P. M.	Eat	Fast	Eat	Fast	Eat	Fast	Eat	Fast
10 P. M.	Eat	Fast	Eat	Fast	Eat	Fast	Eat	Fast

This schedule is not recommended unless you're really determined. You'll see that you are already fasting while you're asleep and continue your fast into the day until the next morning. This can put you close to a 32 hour fast, so it's recommended that you follow the first alternate day schedule, and not the second. However, if you're determined to follow this kind of schedule, then choose to eat 500-600 calories on your fasting days. This can help you deal with the hunger during your fast.

Hopefully, with all these scheduling options, you'll be able to find a type of intermittent fasting that works for you. If you haven't, that's okay! Just adjust one of these schedules to better fit your life. Try not to fast beyond 24 hours at a time, but if you choose to extend your fast, then ensure you eat a small meal to help carry you over your fast. In the next chapter, we will explore some possible meal plans for intermittent fasting.

Chapter 6: Intermittent Fasting and Your Diet

We've talked a lot about the why, how, and when of intermittent fasting. Let's now look at your diet and how it can help you with fasting. There are some diets that are specific to intermittent fasts. For example, the 5:2 method and alternate day fasting both have the option of having small, calorie restricted meals during your fasting days. Most other fasts simply require you to have no food during the fasting window, and during the eating window, eating well balanced meals. The Warrior Diet recommends following a Paleo style diet to bet the most benefits from it. We'll cover all these diet options for fasting. Just remember to eat what works for you.

If you don't want to change your diet, you don't have to. Afterall, intermittent fasting isn't a diet, so you don't have to change if you don't want to. However, if you don't currently have a good diet, a change to a healthier one will help you, with or without intermittent fasting. So, we'll cover some well-balanced meals and nutrition for regular eating without restriction.

5:2 Method and Alternate Day: Calorie Restriction

In the 5:2 method and some alternate day methods, you can eat a restricted diet of 500-600 calories during your fasting window. This helps to curb hunger, and reduce your calorie intake over the course of a week. Your reduction in calories can help with putting your body in ketosis to burn more fat and can also result in more weight loss in comparison to fasting alone. With these two methods, you're getting the best of both worlds and some of the best health benefits of intermittent fasting.

A reduction from 2,000 calories a day to 600 calories can feel quite drastic. So long as you are eating your regular amount of food during your eating days, you'll be okay nutrition and health wise. To get the most out of the calorie reduction, eat a combination of protein and fiber. These two food kinds can help reduce your hunger and keep you fuller, longer.

Depending on how you want to eat throughout your day,

132

your meals are going to vary. Some people divide their allotted calories between two meals. Some people eat one large meal with all the calories for their day in it. Some people simply snack on a variety of low-calorie foods throughout the day. Let's explore some meal types that you could have with calorie restriction. The meals mentioned here will also mention their calories so you can determine how much to eat. You can also use websites and apps to give you more recipe suggestions. Whatever you choose to eat, you need to take the time to either follow the recipe precisely or weigh out your food. This way, you'll have a precise measurement of how many calories you're eating. If you choose to snack throughout the day, we'll provide some snacking options.

It's critically important that you eat at least 1,800 calories on your eating days. This is to ensure that you have enough nutrition to last both your eating day, and your fasting days. You don't want to put too much stress on your body and make it think that you're starving yourself. If you're worried about your diet, talk to a nutritionist to ensure you're eating enough, and getting good nutrients from your meals.

During your fasting window, you could eat 600 calories of marshmallows, but they're not going to provide you with the nutrients you need. So, the ideas mentioned here for your diet contain a good mix of light proteins, fruits, vegetables, and low-fat dairy. There are also a lot of egg recipes, because eggs are amazing, and healthy.

Breakfast ideas

There are a lot of foods out there that are going to provide you with a filling meal, with little calories. These include vegetables and eggs. For breakfast, you want to mix some protein with fiber, and this works perfectly with vegetables and eggs, or fruit and yogurt. The meals in this section are all 300 calories or less. You can follow these ideas to help you choose good breakfast options. If they're not filling enough, add vegetables or fruit that are low in calories. Here are our breakfast recommendations, all for under 300 calories:

134

- An English muffin with cream cheese and spinach. Add some salt and red pepper to spice it up. Follow the regular serving size of cream cheese to keep the calories low.

- One apple, sliced up, and peanut butter. An apple is about 120 calories, so adjust the peanut butter amount to make up 300 calories.

- Vegetables, egg, and feta cheese frittata. Choose a low-fat variety of cheese to reduce calories. Many vegetables like zucchini are low in calories, so you could probably use a quarter zucchini and one egg per serving in the frittata.

- One cup of whole-grain cereal, with one cup of milk and fruit on the side. Choosing a whole grain cereal will help get you some good fiber. The milk is your protein.

- Oatmeal with fruit is another tasty and wholesome option. If you want to add some sugar to it, then adjust the other calories in the meal. You can also make your oatmeal with water or milk. Just adjust to accommodate your calorie intake accordingly.

- Two scrambled eggs with one piece of whole grain toast. Add some butter to your toast but check your portion size to keep the calories low. Margarine isn't recommended because it's not a healthy fat and doesn't provide you any health benefits.

- One slice of whole grain bread with peanut butter and topped with sliced bananas.

While you eat these meals, or any other meals you choose, make sure that you keep a record of how your body reacts to these meals. Do they help alleviate your hunger during a longer fast? Do they make you feel uncomfortable? Just be mindful of what you eat and how it makes you feel while eating these very low-calorie meals.

Lunch and dinner ideas

These two meal times are combined for this section simply because many of the meals are good for lunch or dinner. Pretty straightforward. These meals also try to combine protein and fiber so that you won't be too hungry. Eat of these meals are about 300 calories, and a lot of them are soup and salad! Soup is a great way to get your nutrients in an easily portioned meal. Salad is also fantastic because you can add a lot of leafy greens which are all very low-calorie vegetables. They keep you feeling full, but also provide you with essential nutrients.

- A jacket potato with salsa, sour cream, and perhaps a smidge of cheese. Cheese is delicious, so don't overdo it. Add some chives to give a bit more flavor.

- Fresh rolls with shrimp and a lot of vegetables. Vegetables that work in fresh rolls are spinach, sliced red peppers, sliced cucumbers or radishes. Use them individually or all together for some excellent flavor. Add some sauce on the side, like soy sauce or peanut sauce to dip your fresh rolls in. Avoid sauces full of sugar.

- Onion and potato pancakes with a side salad. This meal doesn't provide a lot of protein, so you can add a boiled egg to your side salad to help with that. But that's more calories.

- One baked chicken thigh with potatoes and swiss chard. Swiss chard can be bitter, so if this isn't a flavor profile you like, substitute with another cooked, leafy green. This meal is really filling and an excellent combination of protein and fiber.

- Winter squash and silken tofu soup. It sounds strange, but silken tofu is perfect for soups and smoothies. In this recipe, cook the squash first with your flavorings and broth, then blend it with tofu. You'll have a perfect protein and fiber combination.

- Pork ragu and polenta. This meal is very

comforting and yet can provide you with good protein and fiber, plus a lot of flavor. Just check your portion sizes to ensure you're eating the right amount.

- Chicken and orzo soup. Add a lot of vegetables to the soup to provide you with more fiber.

- Cheese and broccoli soup. This doesn't sound low calorie, but it can be if you reduce how much fat you put into it. Use chicken or vegetable broth, skim or 1% milk, and only a few ounces of cheese. This will help keep the calories down and will also provide you with a delicious, warming soup.

Salads are also a great option for lunch or dinner. The key here is to have a lot of leafy greens and watch your extras. It's very easy to go overboard with a salad. Sometimes dressings can also be full of calories. You could make your own dressing by combining an oil with an acidic ingredient. For example, olive oil and lemon juice make a beautiful dressing. So does red wine vinegar and olive oil. Choose your dressing wisely and keep your toppings down. Adding protein and other toppings can provide you with a fuller meal, while also satisfying your taste buds. Some protein choices you can add to salad include shredded chicken, shrimp, tuna, beans, hard-boiled eggs or cooked tofu. All of this can satisfy the protein plus fiber combination which will tide you over your fast. Other toppings could be avocado, cheese, nuts, or seeds. While these are all delicious, you'll need to keep your portion sizes in check since it can easily exceed your calorie requirements. Nuts for example are very calorie dense. So, go easy with these kinds of toppings. Here are some salad ideas for your fast:

- Scallops and watercress. Watercress is a good option if you're bored with lettuce or spinach. You could also add crumbled bacon onto your salad for more flavor if you want to.

- Steak and arugula salad. Again, arugula is a good alternative to regular leafy greens in a salad. Arugula is perfect and slightly spicy, giving you a lot of flavor. For more flavor, add some shaved parmesan.

- Grilled corn and pepper salad with shrimp. This salad has no leafy greens, but you can add some to get a more filling lunch or dinner.

- Chickpea, cucumber, and tomato salad. Add some red onion for additional flavor if you want to. If the protein isn't enough for you, replace it with some shredded chicken.

- Caprese salad. This salad is basically mozzarella cheese and sliced tomatoes. Check how much mozzarella you use to make sure you don't go overboard.

Snacking ideas

Having one or two large meals in your day may not be your chosen style. In this case, you should consider snacking over the course of the day to stave off hunger. Your snacks could be large, or simply things to munch on. So long as you're not exceeding 600 calories on your fasting day, you should be okay. Make sure you that you keep a record of how many calories you're eating in your day, by tracking on an app or journal. Here are some snacking ideas for your reduced calorie days.

- Turkey slices and cheese slices. Try to keep it to two slices of deli turkey and two slices of deli cheese. Add some crackers or half a pita. Some sliced cucumbers and carrots can also go beautifully with it.

- Various colored grape tomatoes, two hard boiled eggs, and some wheat crackers. The number of crackers and type of crackers you choose depends on how many calories each is. Make sure you check carefully and eat the right amount.

- Sliced cucumbers and radishes. You can dip them in a little plain yogurt or hummus for some protein.

- Roasted carrots. They're delicious, so nothing else

is really needed unless you want to add more flavor.

- A handful of nuts. Since nuts are calorie dense, keep their number low.

- Half a cup of frozen yogurt. The perfect dessert that also provides some protein.

- A package of plain popcorn. Popcorn is high in fiber and very filling. You won't need to eat a lot and 100 calories worth of popcorn will fill you up. If you want to add flavors, adjust your calorie count accordingly.

- A medley of fruits. This is just a fancy name for some sliced up fruits to munch on. Some good options are clementine segments, sliced apples, strawberries, and sliced kiwi. They're delicious together or on their own.

- A cup of watermelon. Watermelon is a great snack. It provides so much hydration, but also some key vitamins and electrolytes.

- A grapefruit cut in half. This is a perfect tart dessert. If you want to, sprinkle a little sugar on it for added sweetness.

- Low fat yogurt cup and a handful of blueberries. Yogurt can be really filling and satisfying when you're hungry. Try to avoid ones that have fruit on the bottom since they have a lot of sugar in them. Instead, get a reduced sugar variety, or even eat it plain.

- Vegetable plates. You often find these when you go to a party. Having a plate of carrots, broccoli, sliced bell peppers, and celery can be an excellent snacking option. They'll keep you full but with very few calories.

- String cheese. If cheese is what you crave the most, this can help satisfy you. String cheese isn't a lot of calories and is an excellent source of dairy and protein.

When you choose to snack, you still need to count your

calories. Don't gorge until you're full just because all of these are low calorie snacks. A lot of low-calorie items add up to significant calorie gains very quickly. This can derail your goals for weekly calorie reduction. So, make sure you measure how much you eat and keep a record of it.

Warrior Diet: Paleo

The food for the warrior diet is different than the food requirements for the 5:2 method and the alternate day method. The warrior diet doesn't require any calorie reduction at all. In also doesn't really have restricted foods. However, a lot of people recommend following the paleo diet while also doing the warrior diet. Since the paleo diet is healthy, this recommendation isn't really going to harm you. Just remember to eat enough nutrients during your four-hour window to remain healthy.

The paleo diet is one based on our ancestors' lives. It

recommends eating foods that were similarly available in antiquity. So, there is a heavy emphasis on protein like seafood, eggs, and meat. It also emphasizes fruits and vegetables, nuts and seeds, and healthy fats. The paleo diet doesn't allow most grains, sugars, legumes or dairy. Afterall, these were based on heavy agriculture and processing. In general, unprocessed food is recommended over processed foods. So, if it's anything that has been processed, it should be avoided while on the paleo diet.

Since there isn't a calorie restriction when following the warrior diet, the calories will not be included, or really considered, in the foods mentioned in this section. These food options are paleo and will provide you with good nutrition. Just ensure you are getting enough variety to maintain your nutrition. So, don't eat way more protein than any other food group. Mix it up. While grains are prohibited in paleo diets, you can adapt it to fit your lifestyle better. Some people who follow paleo eat rice as their grain.

Breakfast ideas

Depending on your fasting schedule, you may not have a typical breakfast. Afterall, you might just break your fast at 6pm instead of 6am However, the meals can be the same or similar. Remember, before eating this breakfast meal, have something small a couple minutes before, just to readjust your body to eat again after a 20 hour fast. Here are some ideas for your breakfast meal:

- Egg and vegetable frittata. If you need to add oil, use coconut oil or avocado oil. Use a variety of vegetables to give you some different vitamins. You could add spinach, broccoli, and bell peppers. Or tomatoes, onions, and garlic. It will be delicious either way. Add a side of fruit, or a side salad to complete the meal.

- Bacon and eggs — a classic American breakfast. Bacon is allowed in the paleo diet and can provide needed flavor to any meal. Use the bacon fat to cook your eggs or discard the fat and cook your eggs in olive oil.

- Hard-boiled eggs with a cooked spinach and bacon salad. Since this is cooked, it's not really a salad, but it is quite delicious. Add some chives or onions for additional flavor.

If none of these appeal to you, you could always find some other recipes online. Fruits and vegetables are always a good breakfast option. A fruit salad with sunflower seeds can be a perfect break from eating eggs in the morning.

Lunch and dinner ideas

Because you only have a small eating window in the warrior diet, it's hard to really have three large meals. It's more likely that you'll have two meals, or just graze during the four hours. So, in this section lunch and dinner are combined. There will also be some recommendations for 'grazing,' or eating small bits consistently. Whichever path you choose, there are a lot

148

of good food options following a paleo diet.

- Chicken salad and grapes. This may sound a little strange, but chicken salad is wonderful with grapes. You can even add some nuts with it for added texture. If you're eating a paleo version with grains, then having some whole-grain toast with the chicken salad.

- Egg salad. In case you're not bored with eggs, then egg salad can be a delicious meal. Add salsa or guacamole to add some flavor. A side salad can provide some additional nutrients and help you remain full.

- Burgers wrapped in lettuce or without any wrapping. Burgers are a great meal. You just can't eat the bun when following the paleo diet. However, if you want to add grains to your meal, then choose a whole wheat bread with your burger. Whether you have a bun or not, add onions, and other vegetables to your burger. If you want to add something with an amazing taste, then dry some tomatoes in the oven and add them to your burger. Dried tomatoes have an intense flavor which can add something to your meals.

- Salmon and vegetables. Grilled or fried salmon is a great nutrient full meal. Add a side of cooked leafy greens like chard, spinach or arugula to add more nutrients. The fiber from the vegetables can help you remain full during your fasting period.

- Grilled chicken and salsa. Sliced grilled chicken and salsa served on a bed of vegetables can stand in for eating fajitas. Some vegetable options could be grilled onions and peppers, or something like asparagus.

- Steak stir-fry. This can be served with rice, if you're allowing grains as a part of your diet. Choose a steak that you can thinly slice and won't be tough when you cook it. Also slice up some vegetables for your stir fry. Zucchini, asparagus, and corn are good options. Cook it all in coconut oil. Added coconut aminos can give you nice flavor.

- Fresh rolls wrapped in rice 'paper.' This only works if you're allowing grains in your diet. But you can have Vietnamese style fresh rolls that are all wrapped in rice paper. Add some vegetables like peppers and cucumbers to the wrap and top with fish, and an avocado, then wrap it all up.

- Steak with sweet potatoes. This will be very filling. Having sweet potatoes with steak will give you a good mix of protein and fiber, without having to rely on grains. You can do the same combination with chicken and roasted potatoes or fish and potatoes. Add a side salad with arugula for a bit of spice.

If you want to eat constantly during your four hours, instead of having a large meal, then choose items that are whole and unprocessed. Here are some ideas:

- Raw fruits. Nearly any fruit is edible on the paleo diet. So, eat the ones you love the most. You should eat a lot of fruits and vegetables to give you the necessary fiber for your diet.

- Raw vegetables. Just choose the ones you like! Most vegetables are allowed on the paleo diet. Just don't eat legumes like beans and lentils.

- Nuts like pistachios, pecans, and almonds. Most nuts are welcome in a paleo diet, but some are not. Peanuts for example are classified as a legume, so they can't be eaten on a paleo diet.

- Seeds like pumpkin seeds, sunflower seeds, and flax seeds. Seeds are a great snack. You can even turn them into a dessert. You can mix chia seeds, honey, and coconut milk for a delicious 'pudding.' The chia seeds soak up the milk and turn gelatinous, creating a nice dessert.

- Trail mix. Mix up some trail mix with seeds, nuts, and a little chocolate. Dark chocolate that is 70% cocoa is paleo and can give you that little bit of sweetness you're missing.

- Meat or Plant-based Jerky. If you like salty foods, then jerky can be a good paleo option. Just make sure you drink enough water to make up for the salt.

- Hard boiled eggs. Yes, here they are again. Eggs are excellent foods for snacking!

While on the warrior diet, you can eat paleo foods or just follow a regular well-balanced meal. Either way, you'll only have four hours to eat all your required calories, so make sure your meals are nutritious.

Maintaining Well-Balanced Meals

When following a fast, it's important that you're getting the right nutrition, as I've mentioned several times before. If you don't want to follow a specific diet, then aim for healthy, wholesome foods. A good way of doing this is having a well-balanced meal.

Most of us have learned what a healthy meal constitutes

in school. It was drilled into us during health class, possibly pointed to in biology class, and repeatedly mentioned by the school nurse. But most of us don't eat well-balanced meals. We instead eat what's convenient. With so many easy to find restaurants, food can be at our fingertips. Most of that food isn't healthy, and while it can be difficult for some Americans to find healthy foods, if you have them available to you, then choose wholesome foods, rather than fast foods.

If you have difficulty figuring out what makes a well-balanced meal, you can explore some of the resources provided by the U.S. Health Department. They even have a website dedicated to showing how to portion your meals and include all the food groups during your day. The website can offer you customizable meal plans that will give you nutritious meals and can provide other resources so that you can make the best meal decisions for your body type.

When you have a well-balanced meal, it means that you're eating a bit from at least three different food

154

groups. The food groups are fruits, vegetables, grains, proteins, and dairy.

Fruit is...well...fruit. It's self-explanatory. While you want to eat some fruit each day, you're not going to eat as much as you do vegetables. Fruits can be high in sugar, so choose fruits that aren't as high and eat those more frequently. Try a variety of different kinds of fruit because they can each contain different vitamins and nutrients. So, pick and choose, and don't stick with the same fruit every day. Despite what they say, an apple a day doesn't keep the doctor away. Instead, mix up your fruit choices.

The vegetable family includes a lot of variety. Think pumpkins, corn, broccoli, onions, and beans. All of these are part of the vegetable group. They're also one of the largest families of food you should eat during your day. In general, at least one-third or half of your plate should be vegetables. Just like with fruit, you want to mix up your vegetables because they each provide a different type and number of vitamins. For example, yellow pumpkins can give you way more vitamin A than many other veggies. So, mix it up.

Grains are a large food group and the family consists of food produced by a grain plant. Some grain plants include wheat, bran, rye, rice, oats, and sometimes corn. All of this is then processed into other foods like bread, oatmeal, polenta, tortilla's, cereal, etc. All of these are a part of the grain food family. Grains should also be a large part of your meal. About one third of your plate will be grains. Whole grains are a better option than other types. Think whole-wheat bread vs. white bread. Choose brown rice over white rice. These types of grain contain more nutrients.

The protein family has a variety of different items in it. It can contain lean meats that are unprocessed, seafood, beans, nuts, and tofu. Some lean meats are lamb, beef, and pork. Sausages, hot dogs, and salami are considered processed and less healthy. You should eat these only in small quantities. But lean meat itself is quite healthy and you should eat about seven servings in a week.

Seafood is another great choice and you should have at least two servings in your week. Seafood includes fish, shrimp, scallops, octopus, etc. Beans, nuts, and tofu are other kinds of protein. They are all plant based and are excellent alternatives to meat or seafood. You should try to have some meatless/plant-based foods during your week and beans can give you an alternative that will keep you full.

The dairy family is our last food group. It consists of animal products like milk, eggs, cheese, and yogurt. When you choose a dairy item, it should be a low-fat variety. Full fat yogurt can be very healthy and provide you with essential vitamins and probiotics. Dairy should only be a small percentage of your daily dietary consumption.

When choosing well-balanced meals, try to avoid heavily processed foods and fast foods. These can be full of sugar, carbs, and fats that aren't healthy for you. However, eating out every now and again is completely fine. Just don't make it a daily habit. Other foods like processed meats, alcohol, fatty foods, and 'junk' foods should be limited so that they do not take up a huge portion of your weekly eating.

While you fast, you want your food choices to give you the best balance of nutrients. So, following a well-balanced meal will help you maintain your weight, or even promote weight loss depending on what your diet was like before you started fasting. While you could eat all the right nutrients, you might still be sabotaging yourself with your portion sizes. So be aware of the portion size as well as the nutrients in each of your meals. Below, we'll explore some possible meal ideas that are well-balanced.

Breakfast ideas

When you break your fast, try to eat a combination of protein and fiber to keep you full. It will also help you recover, if you decided to work out before fasting. Make sure that your keeping a record of what you eat so that you can check to see how your body responds to different foods after a long fasting period. Some people can have a negative reaction to eating certain foods after breaking their fast, so stay mindful about what you're eating and check in with yourself regularly to see if you're reacting badly to something you ate. Here are some great well-balanced breakfast ideas.

- Whole-grain English muffins with eggs, butter, and spinach. Add a side of fruit like mixed berries or a banana. This meal covers four food groups: grains, protein, dairy, and vegetables.

- Oatmeal with sunflower seeds, diced apple, and a bit of yogurt. This meal has items from four food groups. The yogurt is your protein, and the oatmeal is your fiber and grain. So, this meal will keep you fuller than just eating toast alone.

- Whole grain bread with peanut butter or a nut butter alternative. Add some fruit on the side or on the sandwich itself. Consider blueberries on top of peanut butter and toast. Or bananas. Bananas and peanut butter are magic.

- Yogurt with fruit, nuts, and some crumbled granola. This meal provides you four different food groups. This is heavier in dairy, so you would want to have less dairy in the rest of your day. Alternatively, you can substitute dairy for non-dairy milk options as well if you are dairy-intolerant. Increase how much fruit you add if you want to have a fiber rich breakfast.

- Cheese omelette with diced peppers, onions, and broccoli. Eat it with a side of toast if you want to add a grain.

A lot of the meals listed here have items from four food groups. You don't have to do that for your meals. These are just recommendations. In general, just make sure you combine a protein and fiber to keep you full. An example would be having Raisin Bran cereal (fiber) with a cup of 2% milk (protein).

Lunch ideas

With lunch, try to make a good portion of your meal vegetables. This will help you meet your daily vegetable serving and give you a good amount of nutrients and vitamins. A good option is having a salad for lunch, but this can be unwilling. So, add some protein and one other food group. All of this can help you have a satisfying lunch while fasting. Here are some lunch ideas.

- Cobb salad with a mix of leafy greens, roasted beets, tomatoes, crumbled blue cheese, and hard-boiled eggs. If you don't want to eat eggs with your lunch, substitute them for canned beans. Black beans and roasted chickpeas are good alternatives.

- Shrimp bowl with brown rice, lime flavored shrimp, sliced tomatoes, and avocado salsa. This meal provides you with your protein and fiber. It also gives you some tasty foods with avocado salsa and lime-flavored shrimp. If you're warming it up at work, check in with your coworkers, just in case the scent of seafood is off putting for anyone else around the office.

- Roasted chicken, with arugula salad and roasted new potatoes. This meal is one that you could also have for dinner. You could bring the leftovers for lunch. Whichever way, it will be filling and be a tasty alternative to eating out for lunch.

- Jacket sweet potato with corn salsa, sour cream, and black beans. This vegetarian lunch provides you with a lot of protein from the beans and sour cream. If you don't want to eat sour cream, then replace it with plain Greek yogurt.

- Five bean chilies. This will have a lot of protein and fiber from the beans, as well as a good amount of vegetables from the tomatoes, onions, and garlic in the chili.

If these don't appeal to you, then find some recipes

online that look interesting. Don't feel limited by what's listed here. There are so many recipes out there that can help you choose healthy options while also being very delicious. Take some time to pick out some things you can cook and eat during the week. This will make your fasting easier if you already have your meals planned out.

Dinner ideas

This is usually your last meal before your fast. So, you want to make it very nutritious and something that will help tide you over your fasting period. If you're going to bed immediately after eating, then choose things that aren't going to disrupt your sleep. Some people feel like dairy before bed gives them nightmares, so if you're one of those people, skip dairy in your dinner. If you're having disrupted sleep but don't know the cause, then check your food journal. What did you eat before bed every night? Perhaps the problem is there. Or perhaps the problem is elsewhere. Having a record of your food choices can help you make the best decisions for your health.

To make your meal planning easier, make enough dinner to bring the extras for lunch the next day. This can help you make fasting easier. You could also plan your meals for the week on the weekends, then spend your time cooking them during your weekend. This way, all your meals are already prepared, and you just must reach into the fridge for one type to eat. Having your meals planned out will help you while you're fasting. It will also reduce and feelings of food obsession, since you'll already have things prepared and won't be constantly thinking of other foods. Here are some well-balanced meal ideas:

- Beef and cheese lasagna. Add vegetables in between the layers for added nutrients. Some great options are sliced eggplant, roasted red peppers, even some spinach. All of them can add to the value of your meal. If this doesn't appeal to you, then eat the lasagna with a side salad, using a variety of vegetables. Keep your portions small since lasagna can have a lot of cheese in it.

- Steamed trout with a side of new potatoes and swiss chard. This is one of my favorite meals. Trout is delicious and full of good antioxidants. It also tends to be less expensive than salmon, making it affordable and accessible. Swiss chard is bitter, and some people don't like it. If it's not your cup of tea, then replace it with other leafy vegetables like collard greens or kale.

- Chicken curry with potatoes and green peas. Depending on how you make your curry sauce, you should have a lot of vegetables already in the curry itself. The spices in curry are very good for you and can provide a lot of nutrients.

- Pumpkin soup with cashews and coconut milk. This is honestly divine. You'll get your protein from the coconut milk and cashews, with the fiber from the pumpkin. It's very smooth and decadent. If this flavor profile isn't for you, try it with chicken broth replacing the coconut milk, and crumbled bacon replacing the cashews. As some thyme to taste.

- Slow-cooked shredded pork tacos. Use roasted pineapple in the tacos and add thinly sliced vegetables like radishes or lettuce. Choose whole wheat or corn tortillas to wrap your tacos, and top with salsa or guacamole.

Try to have at least a couple servings of fish in your week and consider some meatless meals. Eating too much meat is not very healthy, so mix it up. Replace some meat in your favorite recipes with tofu or beans instead.

To conclude this chapter, all these different kinds of foods and meals can help you be successful with your intermittent fast. Choose the type of diet you want to follow for your fast, or don't change your diet at all. The choice is entirely up to you. If you notice that you're gaining weight while on the fast, then look at your diet. It may be the problem. If you're not satisfied with what you're currently eating on your fast, then change your diet! For people who are not following the 5:2 or alternative day method, try to maintain a diet that has at least 1,300 calories during your days. Otherwise you'll be in danger of becoming malnourished. Good luck with your meals on the fast!

Chapter 7: Motivation to Stick with Your Plan

I wish I could tell you that fasting is all sunshine and roses. I wish I could tell you that it's so easy to follow. Unfortunately, it's not. There are going to be days when you look at your cup of coffee and cry because you can't eat anything for another four hours. There are going to be days when you throw yourself at the doors of the local cafe and ogle all the pastries and lattes, knowing that by the time you can eat, the doors will be closed. There will be days when all your friends are out drinking and partying, and your eating window just ended. Basically, there are going to be frustrating days, sad days, difficult days, stressful days, and nightmare days where you're going to want to throw in the towel and give up on your fast. These are the kinds of days that you'll need motivation to help you continue your fast. Without the motivation, it's likely that you'll end your fasting period early, not start the next fasting period, or just give up all together.

One key thing you can do to keep yourself motivated is

to remind yourself of the days that were amazing. Think about that day last week, when you had your latte and your boss didn't yell at you. Think about that morning, when your dogs lovingly jumped on the bed and woke you up with millions of kisses. Think about that time that you dropped your scarf on the train and someone found it and returned it to you. The recollection of these good days can help remind you that your days will get better. You can use these reminders on the rough days when you just want to give up on fasting, or the days when you just want to sit on the bathroom floor and cry.

When your days are rough and you have the stress of fasting on top of that, it's likely that you'll break your fast. However, it's important that you continue your fast again in the future, even if you hit some speed bumps along the way. This chapter will cover some points that may help you continue to feel motivated.

Distract Yourself

Sometimes the hunger that comes with fasting can be overwhelming. This is especially true with fasts that require 24 hours of not eating. If you can't seem to stop thinking about food, or if you're just feeling gnawing hunger, then you might want to break your fast early and just eat everything in front of you. Before doing that, see if some distractions will help you maintain your fasts. Some good distractions include work, exercise, and meditation.

Work probably shouldn't be classified as a distraction, but it can be a useful one when you're fasting. Having your mind occupied by something that requires you to be actively engaged is a great way to distract yourself from your feelings of hunger. Many of us have already experienced this. If you've ever been in the 'flow' while working, you've probably skipped meals without realizing it. You may have even come out of flow and realized that hours have gone by and your stomach is growling at you. This realization can help you when you're fasting. You can try to get into a state of flow, but if that is beyond you at that moment, then just get engaged with work. Start a new project or plan. If your work is very active, then get fully engaged with the activity. If your work is passive, then find another way to distract yourself.

One way of distracting yourself is to do some light exercises. Depending on the fast you're following, heavy exercise might be too much. Light exercises on the other hand, can be a great distraction and won't affect you negatively. Light exercises include things like walking and yoga. They aren't high intensity and don't involve too much effort on your part. So, they shouldn't cause you to feel nauseous or faint. Walking outside in nature is a perfect distraction. Instead of walking and focusing on your hunger, focus on things outside of you. Look at the trees, birds, and insects. Observe the other people around you, breathe in deeply, and just walk. Allow your mind to wander, but if it keeps going to your hunger, then refocus on something else. Yoga is another way that you can distract yourself. Because it requires more focus on the positions and your breath, you will quickly find yourself distracted from your hunger.

Use your distractions wisely. While it's okay to distract yourself from feeling hungry, it's not okay to distract yourself from feeling intensely uncomfortable. If you're feeling unwell, then this is a sign to step back from the fast and speak to a doctor. Don't "power through" something that isn't working for you.

Remind Yourself of Your Goals

When you fast, you usually have reasons for why you are choosing to do it. Maybe your goal is to lose weight, maybe it's just gone get healthier in general. Your goals should be personal to you, not something that's mimicry of other people's goals. Think about why you really want to fast. Think about a goal that will really motivate you to continue fasting. Whatever your reasoning, your goals can help you maintain motivation. To help you remember your goals, write them down. You can put them in the same journal you put your food notes in, or you can make a specific fasting journal with your fasting schedule, food notes, and goals all together. Having them written down makes them more concrete and gives you something to look back on when your fast becomes difficult to sustain.

As you start to feel weary of continuing your fast, or if you struggle with the hours without food, then take the time to say your goals. Write them down somewhere so you see them frequently. You can use a dry erase marker and put your goals on your bathroom mirror. That way every day as you start your eating window you can see your goals, and every evening as you bring your eating window to a close, you're reminded of why you're fasting. During the day, when you struggle with your fast, take a moment to repeat your goals to yourself. You can say it like a mantra to help you stay focused and ignore the hunger.

Beyond repeating your goals to yourself, you can create a visual to help embody your goals. You can create a vision board. A lot of people create these boards to help remind them of their goals in many aspects of their lives.

Usually, it's created with cutouts from magazines or printed pictures. Each image represents something specifically to you. If your goal is to buy a house, then you might have a picture of a beautiful house. For fasting, if your goal is to be healthier, then your picture can be anything that embodies the word 'health' to you. It could be people exercising, or even just a mountain with clean air. Your images are unique to you. Once you have your goal images, put them together in a collage and post them somewhere that you'll see your vision board every day. Your office or kitchen, maybe your bedroom, are all good choices.

Finally, if fasting is really getting you down and you don't have your vision board or written goals near at hand, then do a visualization technique. Close your eyes and in your mind, visualize yourself as you have reached your goal. What do you look like? What emotions do you feel? How do you feel physically? How do you feel mentally? Consider all these questions to help you visualize your goal achievement. This can help you remain motivated to fasting, and give you the encouragement to keep going, even after you've broken your fast.

Be Compassionate Towards Yourself

Have you ever notices that the closer we are to someone, the harsher we are to them? Like, our acquaintances see us as these perfect angels, but our friends know that we have a sharp wit, and an even sharper tongue. Our family knows that we don't take no nonsense from anyone and our family gets a big brunt of our anger when we feel miserable. But the person we treat the worst is ourselves. Any slight failure or disillusionment results in us reprimanding ourselves. Comments like, "I'm so stupid" or "Why am I such an idiot?" are things that we say to ourselves. We would never say them to our friends or acquaintances. So, we're insanely harsh to ourselves.

When to hit a snag with fasting, maybe cheat a little with what we eat or skip a fasting period, it's not uncommon for us to have some self-recriminating thoughts. These thoughts aren't beneficial. They often tear us down without providing an area to build ourselves up again. They can be extremely negative and result in us giving up our fasts all together. Instead of sulking with our own thoughts and giving up on our fasts, we should try to practice a little self-kindness.

What would you say to a friend who said they failed at their fast and they're so stupid? Would you agree with them? That's unlikely. It's more likely that you'll try to console them, reassure them that they aren't stupid, and follow up by encouraging them to continue trying. Do the same thing that you would do for a friend but do it for yourself. Instead of saying, "I'm so stupid, I failed," say, "I took a cheat day, and that's okay. I'll get right back into my fasting schedule." Be positive and compassionate towards yourself. We all make mistakes and we all have lapses. Simply learn from your experience, adapt your fasting schedule to accommodate what you've learned, and start fasting again. Don't give up just because of a little bump in the

177

road.

Get Some Support + Bonus 16/8 method

Things are always easier with support. Some of us like to think that we're eagles, living solo among all the turkeys. We want to be free without anyone there to back us up. We don't need them! But this isn't ideal, especially when things are difficult. Sometimes, it's better to be surrounded by turkeys who care about you and will support you. Sometimes it's better to be the turkey because you know you're lovingly supported by your friends and family with you. What I'm trying to say here is that when you struggle with intermittent fasting, having the support of your friends can really make a difference in your success or failure.

If you have some friends who are very supportive of you, make sure they know when you're struggling with your fasting goals. They can probably give you a good shoulder to cry on and may even give you some tips for how to make things easier. If you're very lucky, your friends may join your fast with you. This way, you can keep each other accountable. If they don't want to fast, that's okay too so long as they're supportive of you following your health goals.

If you're truly an eagle, alone in the world, then seek support from online communities. There are a lot of blogs and forums out there, dedicated to intermittent fasting. Join some of them and talk to others who are struggling. Some great forums to join include the Reddit forum on intermittent fasting. There, they post pictures of success, questions about speed bumps, and even give each other motivation. Get involved and you'll have some support too.

To conclude this chapter, fasting is hard, but it can be done with the right support behind you and the motivation to push forward. Keep persevering, keep trying, and only give up if your body can't handle the fast. Even when you make a mistake or take a cheat day (or month), just try again when you're ready. Keep trying.

Chapter bonus: 16/8 schedule

Step 1: Planning Your Eating Schedule

This may be the biggest change that you experience as you transition from other fasting types. If you were previously doing the 14/10 method, then this won't be a huge change, but if you're transitioning from the 5:2 method or the alternate-day method, then you'll need to work on your eating schedule. You only have eight hours to eat during your day, so you need to plan when you'll have your meals. This will help ensure you don't get hangry during your day and you have enough in your system to keep you good during your fast time. Determine how you are going to break your fast and end your fast. Consider when you'll eat during the day and how that will fit into your regular schedule. Also consider how you'll handle special occasions with your friends and family.

Just like it was discussed in the transition for beginners, consider whether you will follow this fast daily or only a couple days a week. You'll reap the most benefits from a daily fast, but it's up to you and your lifestyle.

One thing to consider when making your schedule is following your natural circadian rhythm. This was discussed in detail in chapter 1 and again in the section about transitioning from scratch, but we're mentioning it again in case you skipped that section. Following your circadian rhythm is something to keep in mind for your fasting schedule. Most people have a slump in the middle of the day, around 3:00 p.m. You have the most energy in the morning, so you want to take advantage of your natural circadian rhythm. Then you can time your eating window to start at 7:00 a.m. and end at 3:00 p.m. This will put your body in a better metabolic state and help your body burn more fat than if you eat late at night. This schedule might not work for everyone, especially if you do shift work or if you have a family you're caring for. So, find a schedule that works for you and take advantage of the times you feel naturally more energized in your day.

Finally, ensure that you are also maintaining your own sleep schedule. You'll need to have a set sleeping time and waking time to better time your fast. If you followed the 5:2 method or alternate-day method, this might not have been so important. After all, you could eat regularly every other day, and it didn't really matter how many hours you slept. However, having a set sleep schedule will help you determine how many hours to fast while on the 16/8 method. If you sleep eight hours a night, you will only need to fast for an additional eight hours when you're awake. If you get less sleep, you'll need to adjust your fasting time during the day.

Step 2: Starting Your Transition

Your transition schedule is going to follow the same as the beginner's schedule, except you'll need to start from a day when you've done regular eating. If you're currently following the 5:2 method or the alternate-day method, make sure that you are eating enough calories the day before you start your new fast schedule. Then that night, you can start your fast. Here's the schedule, which is the same for beginners:

In week 1, for the first three days, stop eating an hour before you go to bed and start eating one hour after you wake up. This puts you at a 10-hour fast, with 14 hours to eat. After those first three days, you're going to add an hour before bed and after waking up. So, you'll stop eating two hours before bed and start eating two hours after waking up. This puts you at 12 hours of fasting and 12 hours of eating. Three days later, add another two hours, bringing you up to 14 hours of fasting and 10 hours of eating. Then finally, extend to the full 16 hours of fasting and 8 hours of eating. This schedule is perfect if you're planning on doing the midday eating window or late day eating window. But if you want to do an early morning eating window, then move your fasting hours to before bed. For instance, in the first three days, stop eating two hours before bed. Then the next three days, stop eating four hours before bed. Continue until the last three transition days, where you stop eating six or eight hours before bed.

Both transitions should slowly get you into the full fast and help curb the discomfort you might feel. This will take about two weeks to get to the full fast.

You can jump right into the 16/8 method if you were

previously following the 12/12 method or the 14/10 method. You can jump right into the 16/8 from any other method, too, but you might experience some discomfort from the change.

Step 3: Preparing for Discomfort

Since you've fasted before, you probably know about the discomfort you might feel at the beginning of a new fast. If you're transitioning from a fast that included severe calorie restrictions, like the 5:2 fast, then be prepared for how eating more in a day will change your body. You might feel bloated or some gastric distress. For everyone else who has been fasting without calorie restrictions, just keep in mind that each transition brings its own level of discomfort. You might not have any issues if you're changing from the 14/10 fast to the 16/8 fast, but just be prepared in case. Keep in mind any warning signs that you should talk to a doctor about. Things like dizziness, vertigo, feeling weak, or changes in your heart rate all require you to see your doctor. If you're feeling particularly weak after shifting to the 16/8 method, then make sure that your meals have enough calories and are well-balanced.

Step 4: *Recording Things in Your Journal*

Keep a fasting journal for your 16/8 fast. If you've kept one before, then just add to it with your new fasting plan. Record your new goals, all the changes you're going through, and what you are experiencing with the change in eating schedule. Find areas where you are feeling better with the change and areas where you might be feeling discomfort. It's important to record these instances because you can then go back and determine what might be causing discomfort. Maybe it was a meal you ate or poor sleep the night before. Having a record of your day to day while fasting can help you control how your body is feeling. One thing to record is your meals. You want to make sure you're getting enough calories during the day and that you're feeling full enough that you won't be hungry in the middle of the day.

Typical **Schedule** for the 16/8 method

We've gone over the step-by-step process of transitioning into your fast. We've also looked a bit at making sure you have a clear record of the steps you are taking and how your body is adapting to the fast. Now let's look at some possible schedules for your fast. There is a schedule for your transition period and a schedule that examines what your daily eating times and windows will look like. Here are some additional things to keep in mind before looking at schedules:

- *Your choice of schedule is personal.* Create one based on your work schedule or other circumstances in your life. If you want to have dinner with your family, then use that meal to close out your eating window. Count back eight hours to figure out when your first meal will be.

187

- *Your fasting schedule doesn't have to be set in stone.* Try out different times or change your fasting window for special occasions. You don't want to be limited by your schedule, especially when it comes to your social life.

- A great option for scheduling is to follow the times when you're naturally more awake and aware and end your fast before your natural slumps. Each person has a different internal clock, so determine your schedule based on that. Following your natural circadian rhythm is a good place to start; adapt from there.

Early Eating Schedule

This schedule is a great option because it takes advantage of your circadian rhythm. It also is the ideal time in general to eat because it avoids eating late at night. However, it means that you're going to eat an early dinner, which might not work for everyone. With this schedule, you'll start eating at 7:00 a.m. and end at

3:00 p.m.

Here is how to ease into your fast:

Time	Days 1–3	Days 4–6	Days 7–9	Days 10–12
7:00 a.m.	Wake up Eat	Wake up Eat	Wake up Eat	Wake up Eat
9:00 a.m.				
11:00 a.m.	Eat	Eat	Eat	Eat
1:00 p.m.				
3:00	Snack		Eat	Eat

p.m.				before 3
5:00 p.m.		Eat	Fast	Fast
7:00 p.m.	Eat	Fast	Fast	Fast
9:00 p.m.	Fast	Fast	Fast	Fast
10:00 p.m.	Sleep/fast	Sleep/fast	Sleep/fast	Sleep/fast

Here is your weeklong schedule once you've eased into the fast:

Time	12:00 a.m.– 7:00	7:00 a.m.	11:00 a.m.	2:00 p.m.	3:00 p.m.– 2:00

	a.m.				a.m.
Monday to Sunday	Fast/sleep	Breakfast (either light or the largest meal of the day)	Large meal	Last meal, finished by 3:00 p.m.	Fast/sleep

Midday Eating Schedule

Some people have difficulty with eating first thing in the morning. In this case, you can start your fast later in the day. This fast is ideal for people who want to eat right in the middle of the day. It gives you time to wind down before bed and prepare your body for a time of rest without too much digestion happening while you sleep.

191

It also gives you time to exercise in the morning before you break your fast if you want to.

Here is how to ease into your fast:

Time	Days 1–3	Days 4–6	Days 7–9	Days 10–12
6:00 a.m.	Sleep/eat	Sleep/east	Sleep/fast	Sleep/fast
8:00 a.m.	Eat	Eat	Eat	Fast
10:00 a.m.				Eat
12:00 p.m.	Eat	Eat	Eat	

2:00 p.m.	Snack	Snack		Eat
4:00 p.m.				
6:00 p.m.	Eat	Eat	Eat	Eat before 6:00 p.m.
8:00 p.m.			Fast	Fast
10:00 p.m.	Sleep/fast	Sleep/fast	Sleep/fast	Sleep/fast

Here is your weeklong schedule once you've eased into the fast:

Time	12:00 a.m.– 7:00 a.m.	10:00 a.m.	2:00 p.m.	5:00 p.m.	6:00 p.m.– 12:00 a.m.
Monday to Sunday	Fast/sleep	Breakfast (either light or the largest meal of the day)	Large meal	Last meal, finished by 6:00 p.m.	Fast/sleep

Evening Eating Schedule

This schedule doesn't take advantage of your circadian rhythm, and it might not give you the most benefits in changing glucose and cortisol levels. However, this schedule can work for people who really appreciate social eating or people who work at unconventional hours. You can always eat a bit earlier to change this schedule.

Here is how to ease into your fast:

Time	Days 1–3	Days 4–6	Days 7–9	Days 10–12
12:00 a.m.–6:00 a.m.	Sleep/fast	Sleep/fast	Sleep/fast	Sleep/fast

8:00 a.m.	Fast	Fast	Fast	Fast
10:00 a.m.	Eat	Fast	Fast	Fast
12:00 p.m.		Eat	Fast	Fast
2:00 p.m.	Eat		Eat	Fast
4:00 p.m.	Snack	Eat	Snack	Eat
6:00 p.m.		Snack		
8:00 p.m.	Eat		Eat	Eat

		Eat		
10:00 p.m.		Eat		
12:00 a.m.			Eat	Eat before midnight

Here is your week-long schedule once you've eased into the fast:

Time	12:00 a.m.– 8:00 a.m.	8:00 a.m. – 4:00 p.m.	4:00 p.m.	8:00 p.m.	11:00 p.m.– 12:00 a.m.

Monday to Sunday	Fast/sleep	Fast	Breakfast (either light or the largest meal of the day)	Large meal	Last meal, finished by midnight

These three different schedules give you some options for following your 16/8 fasting schedule. As mentioned before, adapt the schedules to better fit your own daily rhythm and lifestyle. It's ideal if your schedule is consistent, but it doesn't have to be set in stone. If you know you want to celebrate your best friend's promotion at the end of the week, then shift your fasting schedule to accommodate eating with your friends. Remember, fasting isn't a diet; it's just an eating schedule. It doesn't need to be permanent, and there shouldn't be any guilt about shifting your schedule. Since we've now discussed several schedule possibilities and how to ease into them, we'll spend the next couple of chapters looking at food choices and some meal plans.

Conclusion

Well look at that! You've made it to the end of the book. I hope the journey was worth it and that you're now ready to start your intermittent fasting schedule. We've covered many topics within these chapters. You now know the basics of intermittent fasting. You know what it is, and the different types of fasts. You know the myths associated with fasting and the benefits and risks of starting a fast. You know exactly how to transition into your fast and what foods will give you the most advantages while fasting. You also know ways to help you stay motivated.

Intermittent fasting is a great way to take control of your health and weight. I would wholeheartedly recommend it to anyone who is struggling to change their relationship with food. Therefore, I wrote this book! I hope the book has helped you learn more about fasting and I also hope you'll give it a chance. Remember to take it slow and really consider all aspects of fasting before diving in. It's a great opportunity to improve your life so hopefully you'll try it. Good luck with your health and wellness journey!

References

The Editors of Encyclopedia Britannica. (n.d.). Fasting. Retrieved from https://www.britannica.com/topic/fasting

Alhamdan, B. A., Garcia-Alvarez, A., Alzahrnai, A. H., Karanxha, J., Stretchberry, D. R., Contrera, K. J., ... Cheskin, L. J. (2016). Alternate day versus daily energy restriction diets: which is more effective for weight loss? A systematic review and meta-analysis. Obesity Science & Practice, 2(3), 293–302. doi: 10.1002/osp4.52

Anson, R. M., Guo, Z., Cabo, R. D., Iyun, T., Rios, M., Hagepanos, A., ... Mattson, M. P. (2003). Intermittent fasting dissociates beneficial effects of dietary restriction on glucose metabolism and neuronal resistance to injury from calorie intake. Proceedings of the National Academy of Sciences, 100(10), 6216–6220. doi: 10.1073/pnas.1035720100

Azevedo, F. R. D., Ikeoka, D., & Caramelli, B. (2013). Effects of intermittent fasting on metabolism in men.

Revista Da Associação Médica Brasileira, 59(2), 167–173. doi: 10.1016/j.ramb.2012.09.003

Berg, J. M., Stryer, L., Tymoczko, J. L., & Gatto, G. J. (2019). Biochemistry. New York: Macmillan international higher education.

Bjarnadottir, A. (2016, October 12). Alternate-Day Fasting - A Comprehensive Beginner's Guide. Retrieved from https://www.healthline.com/nutrition/alternate-day-fasting-guide#section1

Cox, O. (2015). The Five Food Groups. Retrieved from https://www.eatforhealth.gov.au/food-essentials/five-food-groups

Furmli, S., Elmasry, R., Ramos, M., & Fung, J. (2018). Therapeutic use of intermittent fasting for people with type 2 diabetes as an alternative to insulin. BMJ Case Reports. doi: 10.1136/bcr-2017-221854

Gunnars, K. (2018). The Paleo Diet - A Beginner's Guide Meal Plan. Retrieved from https://www.healthline.com/nutrition/paleo-diet-meal-plan-and-menu#section8

Gunnars, K. (2019, July 22). 11 Myths About Fasting and Meal Frequency. Retrieved from https://www.healthline.com/nutrition/11-myths-fasting-and-meal-frequency#section11

Heilbronn, L. K., Smith, S. R., Martin, C. K., Anton, S. D., & Ravussin, E. (2005). Alternate day fasting in nonobese subjects: effects on body weight, body composition, and energy metabolism. The American Journal of Clinical Nutrition, 81(1), 69-73. doi: 10.1093/ajcn/81.1.69

Keys, A., Brozek, J., Henshel, A., Mickelson, O., & Taylor, H. L. (1950). The biology of human starvation (Vol. 1-2). Minneapolis, MN: University of Minnesota Press.

Klempel, M. C., Bhutani, S., Fitzgibbon, M., Freels, S., & Varady, K. A. (2010). Dietary and physical activity adaptations to alternate day modified fasting: implications for optimal weight loss. Nutrition Journal,

9(1). doi: 10.1186/1475-2891-9-35

Klempel, M. C., Kroeger, C. M., Bhutani, S., Trepanowski, J. F., & Varady, K. A. (2012). Intermittent fasting combined with calorie restriction is effective for weight loss and cardio-protection in obese women. Nutrition Journal, 11(1). doi: 10.1186/1475-2891-11-9

Kubala, J. (2018). The Warrior Diet: Review and Beginner's Guide. Retrieved from https://www.healthline.com/nutrition/warrior-diet-guide#benefits

Martin, B., Mattson, M. P., & Maudsley, S. (2006). Caloric restriction and intermittent fasting: Two potential diets for successful brain aging. Ageing Research Reviews, 5(3), 332–353. doi: 10.1016/j.arr.2006.04.002

Patterson, R. E., Laughlin, G. A., Lacroix, A. Z., Hartman, S. J., Natarajan, L., Senger, C. M., ... Gallo, L. C. (2015). Intermittent Fasting and Human Metabolic Health. Journal of the Academy of Nutrition and

Dietetics, 115(8), 1203–1212. doi: 10.1016/j.jand.2015.02.018

(n.d.). Prediabetes - Your Chance to Prevent Type 2 Diabetes | CDC. Retrieved from https://www.cdc.gov/diabetes/basics/prediabetes.html

Schübel, R., Nattenmüller, J., Sookthai, D., Nonnenmacher, T., Graf, M. E., Riedl, L., ... Kühn, T. (2018). Effects of intermittent and continuous calorie restriction on body weight and metabolism over 50 wk: a randomized controlled trial. The American Journal of Clinical Nutrition, 108(5), 933–945. doi: 10.1093/ajcn/nqy196

Wolff, C. (n.d.). 7 Things Nutritionists Wish You Knew About the Warrior Diet. Retrieved from https://www.rd.com/health/diet-weight-loss/warrior-diet/

Intermittent Fasting Meal Plan

Learn How is possible losing weight just following a sequence of meals. Bonus 5/2 method for beginners studied for women and over 50

Jason White

Introduction

For many, fasting has a bad reputation, with religious connotations surrounding it as a form of penance or self-punishment for wrongdoing. To others, the idea of going without food is considered unrealistic and extremely unsafe. But all these notions are deeply rooted in misconceptions and unfounded fears of starvation or guilt over those around the world who actually can't afford food. Eating is how the body survives, but is not designed to eat every few hours as our normal behavior suggests. Filling your body with food 3 to 6 times every day actually has the ability to diminish your overall physical, mental, and emotional health as you age.

The intermittent power system involves several schemes to choose from, so people have the opportunity to select the type of power that suits them.

Sticking to intermittent fasting is not as difficult as it might seem at first glance. With the right choice, a suitable scheme will not require tremendous willpower and continuously struggle with hunger. Intermittent or every other day nutrition provides all the benefits that fasting brings, first of all, it is healing and rejuvenation. In all nutritional schemes, the fasting period does not last longer than a day. This period is enough for the body to switch to internal nutrition, from a medical point of view, this is not starvation, as it occurs just 24 hours after the last meal.

Efficiency from intermittent fasting depends on the lifestyle that a person leads. In the periods between food breaks, the diet will not be limited by anything. This food system does not imply the separation of products into harmful and useful, permitted, and forbidden. Compliance with intermittent fasting does not require preliminary preparation; restrictions after refusing such nutrition are also not provided.

In this book I will share all that you need to know about Intermittent fasting.

Enjoy reading!

Chapter 1: Intermittent Diet

What is Intermittent Diet

Intermittent diet is a diet that requires a pattern of eating where you move between eating and fasting periods. It focuses on WHEN you should/shouldn't eat and less on WHAT you should/shouldn't eat. For this reason, intermittent fasting is not really a diet in the traditional sense, but a form of eating.

Many people report having more energy when fasting. Although hunger can be a challenge, it is manageable and will gradually become easier as your body adapts to longer periods of fasting.

Besides helping with weight loss, fasting has been shown to reduce blood sugar and insulin levels. Fasting can also increase human growth hormone, improve our brain function, and may even help us to live longer. Studies have indicated that fasting may help to protect against health problems such as cancer, diabetes, and Alzheimer's disease.

How it works

Our body can handle extended periods of not eating. Human bodies have the natural ability to transition between the hunger state and the full state. When we don't eat for a long period of time, the processes going inside our body change. When we eat our body starts to work on digesting it and storing the energy received through the meal. When we are hungry, our body starts to take energy from those stored fats.

When we are fasted for a specific period of time, our blood sugar and insulin levels face a reduction in their levels. It is normal because it pushes our body to thrive from existing resources present inside our bodies. Researches have shown that fasting helps to protect against diseases like heart diseases, diabetes, cancer and Alzheimer's disease.

213

Therefore, when in a fasted state, you shouldn't worry that it will affect your health.

In order to understand how intermittent fasting works, two states have to be understood first. The two states are – the fed state and the fasted state. By understanding these states, we get to know that how our bodies keep functioning well regardless of the fact that our stomachs are empty or full.

Two IF states: Fed Vs. Fasted

In the Fed state, the body is undergoing process of digesting and absorbing food. The state begins when you start eating and can last from three to five hours after that. In fed state, your body shows elevated levels of insulin, and this acts as a signal for your body to store the excess amounts of calories. This storage takes place in the fat cells. During the time with high insulin levels, the process of fat burning comes to a stop and the body shifts towards burning glucose from your last meal instead.

Then a state called post-absorptive state comes, which lasts about 8 to 12 hours after the last meal. After that the body enters the Fasted state. In the Fasted state; body is not processing any meal and the levels of insulin are low. This induces a mobilization of stored body fat presiding inside the body in the fat cells, and starts to burn these fats for providing energy to the body. In this state, the body can burn the fat that was first inaccessible to it during the fed state.

Staying hungry for a specific duration of time helps you with hundreds of things. When you eat a meal, your body is under 'fed state' and is just processing the meal you just ate. After a few hours pass and the food is completely digested, it goes into a mid-stage where you don't feel hungry but you haven't eaten anything else yet. You can call this an intermediate state. After 8 to 12 hours from your last meal, a state comes called 'fasted state' when you feel hungry and you are under a fast. In this state, your body needs to re-gain the fuel to work but it doesn't find

214

any energy being provided to it. So, it starts to look for energy sources inside the body. It starts to go towards the fat cells where fats from your previous meals have been stored. The body is designed to store some amount of fat from every meal in order to regain energy at the time when it is needed. Thus, because of low insulin levels now the body has entered into a fat-burning state and it starts to burn the fats present inside the body. This is beneficial in hundreds of ways. It will not only get rid of the excess fat from you, but will also get rid of any toxins present inside a body.

The toxins can be anything harmful present in your body. It can be dysfunctional cell or a cell that is damaged and is not performing well. Removal of such cells is very necessary when we talk about maintaining health. So, you have to be under the 'fasted state' so that your body can initialize the burn-off state. Intermittent fasting provides you a convenient way to enter into the fasted state and get rid of all excess fats, calories and damaged cells. Many health-practitioners and doctors advise their patients to start fasting for this purpose. They believe that health will improve if they fast because of this quality of intermittent fasting.

How to get started with Intermittent Fasting

The most delicate phase of intermittent fasting is the time when you just start it. That is the time when most people give up on it. If people indeed lose some weight, then they get so excited that they start falling back to their old and unhealthy lifestyles and if they do not get the results they wished for, they too they think that intermittent fasting is a complete waste of time. If you have been doing it for a week and got some results, it is really great and I totally appreciate but in order to reap the full benefits, you need to keep practicing it and make it a lifestyle habit. So, here are some tips that will help you start intermittent fasting the right way.

Break Your Fast with the Right Foods

At the end of a fast, when you eat something after a long time, eating the wrong foods can actually spike up the levels of blood sugar, and so you need to be careful about what you are eating. The same thing happens with the level of insulin in the body because they are never consistent. But intermittent fasting has profound benefits when it comes to lowering the levels of insulin in the body. When there is an elevation in the levels of insulin, that is exactly when the body stops burning fat.

Similarly, if insulin is present in huge quantities in your bloodstream, then it will be highly difficult for your body to burn any fat. Now one of the main aims of engaging in intermittent fasting is so that your body can go into a fat-burning mode. So suppose you have complete an almost perfect fast, but in the end, you break it by consuming the wrong type of food, then all that effort that went into the fast was for nothing and the insulin levels will also start to spike.

So, in order to support the process of fat burning, you need to choose foods that are wholesome, and they should not be processed foods. The insulin levels are very heavily impacted when you consume carbs, so your goal is to stick to foods that are low in carbs. Protein has only a moderate impact but there are certain dairy products that can leave quite the impact. The least amount of impact is left by fats and that is also why the keto diet is encouraged when you are on an intermittent fasting regime.

So, stop indulging in carbs or dairy when you are breaking your fast. Sometimes, people overdo it when they break the fast because they think that they somehow have to compensate for the fasting. But it is not that. Also, you need to remember that you can get carried away easily if you are not focused enough. So, when you eat, limit your calories and stick to the food items that have been mentioned in the previous chapter.

Fast for Longer Periods Once You Are Accustomed to the Process

216

Whenever you fast, the amount of insulin in the blood is lowered. So, that is when the body starts burning fat. Thus, the longer you can fast, the longer you can allow your body to stay in the fat-burning mode. But you should not jump into long fasts right in the beginning. At first, you have to master the protocols mentioned in the short-term fasts, and then you have to move on to the longer ones. Extended hours of fasting can be an entire day or you can also try out the 48-hour fast once the full day fasting becomes easy.

The advice that I give to every beginner is that you should start with the 16/8 method because in this, you will have to fast for a period of sixteen hours, and if you decide to skip breakfast, then more than half the fasting window is spent sleeping. So, the process becomes quite easier. After you have performed the 16/8 method for about a week or so and you are feeling that it is becoming easy for you, start by doing a 20-hour fast daily. This means that the eating window becomes really short and you have to squeeze it to four hours. Even if the timeframe is short, you can have two small meals here.

Once you have mastered this too, then you can practice the Warrior Diet, which was mentioned at the beginning of this book. In simpler words, you will have only one meal every day. When you have reached the expert level, then you can take your fasts to 36 hours or 48 hours. At first, such long fasting periods will seem impossible and that is perfectly normal. You are not supposed to do it once but you have to work your way up there. The more you fast consistently, you will notice that the feeling of hunger has started to become blunt. When you are fasting for longer periods, the limitation on calories is increased and fat burning increases too.

Steer Clear of Artificial Drinks

When people are fasting, especially beginners, have this tendency to reach out for the artificial drinks in the form of diet soda, energy drinks, flavored beverages, or even juices. They think that since these drinks claim to have low sugar content, they won't do any harm. But what they don't understand is that these drinks still contain a huge amount of artificial sweeteners that can harm your health.

In order to keep your body hydrated, the only liquid that you should have is water. And when you are doing intermittent fasting, there is no limitation to the amount of water you can drink. Some other drinks that are allowed during intermittent fasting are tea and black coffee, but there should be no sugar. You can also have herbal teas but the criteria remain the same – there should be no milk or sugar in them. These alternatives can easily be swapped in for a soda or other artificial drinks and you can enjoy your fasting windows.

Keep Yourself Busy

This is truly a very truthful tip because if you want your fast to be successful, then you also have to simultaneously keep yourself busy doing something or the other. It can be anything like pursuing a hobby, engaging in your favorite pastime or even work. You can do anything that will involve not thinking about food. This is one of the best ways in which you can adapt to the process of intermittent fasting. In order to be successful with the process, your task is to develop the right mentality and staying will help you with that and this will also make fasts of extended periods bearable.

If you decide to start your fast-post-dinner, then that sorts out most of the problem. Do you know why? It is because the maximum portion of the time will be spent sleeping. That is why beginners are always advised to start their fast-post-dinner. Now, when you are breaking your fast, if you have the meal at around noon, then it can seem quite a long stretch of time to not do anything and sit idle. This is how you will be getting the cravings. So, you need to figure out a way to fill up your mornings so that you can divert your mind from the thought of food. Do

218

some type of productive work. When you are waiting to break your fast with a meal, the last few hours are really crucial and that is also when people lose their patience and break their fast early.

Have Proper Sleep

Whether you are into intermittent fasting or not, sleep will always be essential for you, and it is a universal truth. When you are asleep, your body works to repair your old and worn-out cells. So, sleeping properly is very crucial. You must also know that when you are sleeping, your body burns a certain amount of calories which is crucial to your weight loss journey. This also helps in giving a boost to your metabolism. The fat burning process will make your body undergo a lot of changes in the fasting window.

When you are doing a fast, sometimes you might have the tendency to overeat, and the biggest contributor to this feeling is stress. There are so many people who engage in stress eating. And the worst part about all of this is that stress eating is never related to healthy foods. The foods that stressful people reach out to are sugary in nature and full of carbs. But you have to understand something here – your stress will not be relieved if you have more carbs. Although they help in the production of serotonin which, in turn, makes people feel calmer. So, people think that carbs will help them cope with stress. But this is actually nothing more than a trap! So, to avoid this and avoid the overconsumption of carbs, you need to build a proper mindset so that you can cope with stress and keep it at bay while you are fasting.

Stay Away from Unsupportive People

When you are starting something new, it is very natural on your part to tell others about it, especially the ones you think you are close to. And then, you also seek their approval on the matter not that it is required but it will simply put your mind at ease. But in most cases, your peers or sometimes even your family members might not like the idea and they might even reject your ideas. This happens quite often. Think about all those times when you had just started a new venture and you simply couldn't stop yourself from telling it to others. But the moment you speak with someone else, they shoot you down. This can discourage you to great extents, and sometimes, the criticism they state might not even be true.

It is difficult to start something new or make certain changes in life. The same goes for intermittent fasting – it is a completely new eating plan, and sticking by it for the long-term can be hard. But once you are fully into it, you are definitely going to feel awesome. Starting is probably the hardest part of it all. You need a lot of willpower to start it and even then, you might have several doubts. Now, in this situation, if a friend or a stranger comes to you and says that your idea of fasting is completely bogus, then imagine the disappointment you would feel. The feelings can be so strong that it can make a person feel depressed.

So, sometimes, intermittent fasting is best when practiced with those who appreciate it, and if you do not have such people in your life, then practice it on your own. Never force anyone to join the journey if they are not willing to. If you usually go out with your friends for dinner, then reserve your fasting window for when you are home or you are not socializing, for example, at night and in the morning. If you do it this way, then you can skip on the process of explaining to others why you are doing what you are doing.

Chapter 2: Benefits of Intermittent Fasting

Weight Loss

The most well-known, and looked for, advantage of intermittent fasting is weight loss. Which is understandable, this may also be the main reason why you yourself approached it in the first place. Yet, you may want to explore the topic since there are a lot more advantages that you may not be acquainted with.

As we get older, our digestion system slows down, approaches to perimenopause or menopause and more fat begins accumulating in areas where we do not need it, and intermittent fasting can help.

Some overweight adults who followed an alternate day intermittent fasting plan lost as much as 13 pounds over about two months. Be cautious in case you may want to attempt this strategy in the beginning, since it has some risks such as, for example, eating too much on the days in which you are not fasting.

Not only does intermittent fasting promote fat loss, you likewise hold muscle bulk while fasting, unlike at all typical diets based on calorie cutting.

Intermittent fasting may promote weight loss through a few ways.

To start with, limiting your meals and snacks to a specific time window may for itself diminish your calorie intake, which can help weight loss.

Intermittent fasting may likewise expand levels of norepinephrine, a hormone and neurotransmitter that can help your digestion to increase calorie consuming for the duration of the day.

Moreover, this eating regime may lessen levels of insulin; a hormone associated with glucose. Diminished levels of insulin can knock up fat consumption and increase weight loss.

Some studies even show that intermittent fasting can enable your body to hold bulk more adequately than calorie limitation, which may expand its appeal. Intermittent fasting may diminish body weight by up to 8% and decline body fat by up to 16% over 3–12 weeks.

Defective Cells Cleaning

Intermittent fasting promotes autophagy, which is how the body disposes of cells that are more likely to get contaminated or being destructive. Faulty cells not performing at the highest level can accelerate aging, Alzheimer disease, and type 2 diabetes.

The spontaneous repairing procedure happens to go full speed ahead as the body does not need to concentrate on food assimilation. It can completely focus on cell repair. This procedure is called autophagy.

Consequently, fasting helps immediately relieve the body and makes it work properly.

This disposal of "broken" cells is like a spring-cleaning for your body. It makes room for healthy cells and expands your health and dynamic quality.

Fasting makes our cells become stronger regardless of weight loss.

Intermittent Fasting May Have Anti-Aging Benefits

Over the time, researchers have been looking at the conceivable health benefits of calorie limitation for a considerable length of time.

A likely hypothesis suggests these health benefits are due to the drop in glucose that results from fasting, which pushes our cells to work more diligently to use different sources of energy.

Some rhesus monkeys fed with only 70% of their ordinary caloric intake have appeared to live longer and shown to be healthier in advanced age. This enemy of aging has also been found in animals that were put on an intermittent fasting diet, shifting back and forth between long periods of typical eating and days where calories were restricted.

What is not clear, however, is the reason why intermittent fasting seems to have an important role in the battle against aging. This matter is muddled by the way most of the studies were done on people, when fasting prompted weight loss. The health benefits of weight loss may be overshadowing other benefits acquired from fasting alone.

One way that our cells can be harmed is when they experience oxidative stress. In addition, forestalling or repairing cell damage from oxidative stress is useful in preventing aging. This stress happens when a higher-than-typical generation of free radicals is present. These stressed particles convey exceptionally receptive electrons.

At the point when one of these free radicals meets another particle, it might either give away or acquire an electron. This can bring about a fast chain response from particle to atom, generating even more free radicals, which can break separated associations between iotas inside significant segments of the cell, like the cell membrane, fundamental proteins, or even DNA. Enemies of oxidants work by moving the required electrons to balance out the free radicals before they can do any harm.

In spite of the fact that fasting appears to enable our cells to fight harm from this procedure, it is not precisely clear how that occurs.

Free radicals can be created by inadequately working mitochondria (the powerhouses of the cell). The switch between eating regularly and fasting makes cells briefly experience lower-than-regular levels of glucose, and they are compelled to start utilizing different sources of less promptly accessible energy, like unsaturated fats. This can make the cells turn on endurance procedures to evacuate the unhealthy mitochondria and replace them with healthy ones over time, subsequently lessening the creation of free radicals in the long term.

The cells may react by expanding their levels of oxidants' common enemies to fight against free radicals' creation. In addition, albeit free radicals are usually considered dangerous due to their capacity to harm our cells, they may be significant warning signs for our body.

According to another Harvard University study, intermittent fasting can keep our body more youthful, lengthen our life expectancy, and improve our overall health. Some studies have indicated that intermittent fasting offers no benefits over every day dietary limitations. However, the studies have discovered that it is connected to longer life expectancies.

Breast Cancer Recurrence Prevention

A more extended time of fasting is a decent technique to decrease bosom malignant growth recurrence. An investigation of bosom malignancy survivors who didn't eat for any event 12 and half hours overnight showed a 36 percent decrease in the danger of their bosom disease returning.

Intermittent fasting can help your body with resisting the advancement of the disease. The moment we fast, blood glucose levels decline, and the body begins to utilize our fat stores. This secures against the improvement of malignancy in a few different ways:

- Being overweight expands the danger of creating a wide range of types of disease, by getting in shape through intermittent fasting, we can decrease our malignant growth risk.

- Fasting triggers a change from development to repair. When our body changes to repair mode (autophagy), any harmed cells or parts of cells are stalled, and their bits reused to make new, well-working cells. This especially influences cells which may turn harmful.

- Fasting can likewise diminish the amount of the hormone Insulin-like Growth Factor 1 (IGF-1), which is considered related to an expanded malignancy hazard. A few people appear to have especially high IGF-1 levels, and it seems to exist an unbalanced number of malignancy patients with high IGF-1 levels

- The decline in blood glucose prevents malignant growth cells from fuel. Malignant cells, for the most part, cannot utilize fats or ketones for fuel, they just utilize glucose, thus, though normal cells can be perfectly fine with fats or ketones, the diseased cells are famished and cannot develop.

Lower Risk of Developing Type 2 Diabetes

Type 2 diabetes frequently creates in people over the age of 45. The Centers for Disease Control and Prevention report that more than 30 million Americans have diabetes (around 1 out of 10), and 90%-95% of these have type 2 diabetes.

Type 2 diabetes can create when your cells do not react properly to insulin. Insulin is a hormone secreted in the intestine by the pancreas, which permits cells to assimilate and utilize glucose (sugar) as energy.

In the event that you become insulin resistant, your cells are not open to insulin and cannot process glucose. Sugar at that point develops in your circulatory system, which can be dangerous. Altogether for your body to get the glucose out of the circulation system, it stores it as fat.

Fasting seems to be related to decreases in glucose and upgrades to insulin effectiveness.

Fasting could offer protection against type 2 diabetes by decreasing the fat storage around the pancreas, German specialists have said.

Has recently been discovered that Intermittent Fasting is able to lower HbA1c (glycated hemoglobin) in people with type two diabetes, just as promoting weight loss. Overweight mice conditioned to be at risk of type 2 diabetes showed a gander at the effect that confining meals at specific times had on fat in the pancreas.

Aggregations outside the fat tissue, for example in liver, muscles, or even bones, negatively affect these organs and the whole body.

Boosted and Increased Brain Health

Fasting can soothe cerebrum irritation. Irritation is related to neurological conditions, for example, Alzheimer's disease, Parkinson's disease, and stroke.

Many fasting related effects such as protein sparing, decrease of irritation, autophagy, and increment of BDNF (Brain-derived neurotrophic factor) creation, advantage our cerebrum. From one viewpoint, they decrease the risk of harm to synapses by, for instance, reducing inflammatory reactions. Then again, they additionally favor an appropriate mind work, by advancing cell repair and adding to the arrangement of new synapses and associations between them, in this way encouraging correspondence inside the cerebrum. BDNF specifically increases this structured procedure, and its shortage right now has been connected to psychological issues during aging, for example, dementia. So intermittent fasting has a neuroprotective effect and along these lines promotes a healthy aging.

Improved Heart Health

Fasting can prompt a decrease in pulse, heart rate, cholesterol, and triglycerides in people and animals.

Hard to determine what affects fasting has on your heart health because numerous people who routinely fast frequently do as such for health. Therefore, these people, for the most part, tend to not smoke and have a healthy lifestyle, which can diminish heart ailment chance.

In any case, some investigations have shown that people who follow a fasting diet tend to have better heart health over people who do not. This might be because people who routinely fast show restraint over what number of calories they eat and drink, and this conduct may convert into weight control and better eating decisions when they are not fasting.

Fasting and better heart health may likewise be connected by the manner in which your body processes cholesterol and sugar. Ordinary fasting can diminish your low-density lipoprotein, or "bad" cholesterol. It is also believed that fasting may improve the way in which your body processes sugar. This can decrease your danger of putting on weight and help treating diabetes, which are both risk factors for a heart ailment.

Self-Healing

When you are continually eating, you are not giving your body and your cells the time they need to rest. They need this time to repair themselves, or to dispose of those cells that may get tainted or destructive.

Consider your poor stomach continually working. Give it a rest!

The repair procedure happens to go ahead full speed as the body does not need to concentrate on the absorption of food. Therefore, it can completely focus on cell repair. This procedure is called autophagy.

This way, fasting helps with restoring your body and makes it work appropriately.

One significant advantage of Intermittent Fasting is that you can focus on tasks better and finish a significant segment of your assignments while in the fasting state.

Insulin resistance happens when you continually have high glucose levels. This prompts the powerlessness of your body to follow up on the sugar content in the blood and separate it.

The point when you take up intermittent fasting, it encourages you to monitor your glucose level.

This condition is also activated by elements like high blood pressure, sedentary lifestyle, inheritance factors, ill-advised diet, or excessive body weight.

In any case, other than all the benefits, there are other things to consider. First is the fasting stage that causes the creation of leptin and ghrelin – the appetite hormones. Nevertheless, women over 50, after some time needed to get used to intermittent fasting, report feeling less ravenous over the long term.

The second point is that intermittent fasting is not recommended for pregnant women. Also, in case a woman who fasts should neglect to take in enough calories, she may have some fruitfulness issues. In any case, if done correctly, there's no reason to worry. In the wake of losing, some overweight women may even improve their fruitfulness.

Chapter 3: Exercises to be followed in Intermittent Fasting

The thread that runs through both resistance and cardio training, particularly when it comes to optimal weight loss, is intensity. Simply put, it means the amount of effort put in.

There are three intensity levels when it comes to exercising – low, moderate and high. The optimal intensity is moderate.

So how do you find out your current exercise intensity level? The most straightforward and relatively accurate way of doing so is called the talk test. After exercising for a couple of minutes, try talking as you continue exercising. If you can still carry on a very normal conversation with no effort whatsoever, it means you're exercising at low intensity, which means it's too easy to burn any significant amount of calories. If you can barely talk or carry on a conversation normally, huffing and puffing throughout, your intensity is high, i.e., too hard. If you can still carry on with a normal conversation, but with some effort or strain in breathing or talking, that's moderate intensity – the perfect intensity for optimal fat burning. Moderate intensity must be maintained for a specific period. Otherwise, it won't help you burn significant calories for weight loss. Exercise for too long puts you at risk of losing muscle mass and for too short a period, at risk of being unable to burn many calories. The optimal window is between 20 to 45 minutes of moderate intensity exercise.

Follow the simple exercising tips given in this chapter to speed up the process of weight loss.

Not only can you use fasting as a great nutrition strategy, but you can also use it to help maximize fat loss in the gym. There are a couple of different ways to take advantage of this. The first way is by being in a fasted state when you work out. All you need to do is work out in the morning or early afternoon before you've eaten anything.

When you work out in a fed state, your body will use the glycogen in your body as fuel for energy. However, when you work out fasted, your body will be glycogen depleted. This means that your body won't be able to tap into your glycogen stores for energy, it'll have to go somewhere else. Guess where that somewhere else is? Your fat stores!

So by working out in a fasted state, your body will become more efficient at using fat for energy instead of carbs. The second thing you can do to maximize fat loss from working out is delay eating after your workout. The media has done a good job of making us think we must immediately consume protein after a workout or else it was a waste. Research shows that your body won't lose muscle if you don't eat protein within 45 minutes of your workout.

Whenever you work out, your body's growth hormone levels will increase (11). This growth hormone will help to protect your muscle and increase fat burning. However, if you eat right after you finish a workout, your growth hormone levels will be blunted and insulin levels will increase. For this reason, you'll want to delay eating anything after finishing a workout for 1-2 hours.

Eating more calories won't help you lose more weight. Yet when it comes to eating after a workout, people act like they're immune to gaining fat from these extra calories. "I hit it hard in the gym today, I deserve a large milkshake!" No, you don't.

Imagine you go to the gym and burn 300 calories. Then, immediately after your workout, you consume a 350-calorie post workout protein shake. Now you've completely wiped out all of the calories you burned from the workout, plus you ate an additional 50 calories! It's ok to eat a meal after working out if that's when you would normally eat anyway.

Don't go out of your way to eat extra calories for the sake of a post workout shake—it won't help you burn more fat! You might be weary

230

of working out fasted if you usually workout in a fed state. Give it a try for 1-2 weeks to give your body a chance to adapt to it. Once you do, you should notice that you have more focus and intensity in the gym.

Here's a good beginner's workout plan you can do if you're unsure of what to do in the gym (a more advanced workout will be provided later on in the book):

This regimen consists of 3 full-body weight workouts per week. You'll complete the same workout every time you go to the gym. You can set up your workout schedule in one of the following ways:

Monday: Workout

Tuesday: Rest

Wednesday: Workout

Thursday: Rest

Friday: Workout

Saturday: Rest

Sunday: Rest

Or

Monday: Rest

Tuesday: Workout

Wednesday: Rest

Thursday: Rest

Friday: Rest

Saturday: Rest

Sunday: Rest

As a beginner, full-body workouts will provide you with many benefits:

- You'll burn more calories from your workouts.

- You'll gain strength and muscle faster since you'll be stimulating your muscles more frequently.

- You'll have better nervous system recovery because you won't train on consecutive days.

- You'll develop perfect form on key lifts faster because you practice them more often.

Essentially your body has never been exposed to this stimulus (i.e. weightlifting) before. Therefore, you can take advantage of what some people call "newbie gains." And by increasing the frequency at which you stimulate your muscle groups, you can speed up the process.

Chapter 4: Shopping List for Intermittent Fasting Diet

Grocery shopping might seem like a chore, but it is quite important. Before you decide to head out, you need to make a list of all the groceries that you need. You don't need any junk food or unhealthy foods stored at home if you are trying to eat healthily. So, the first thing that you need to do is clear your pantry off all the food items that aren't healthy. Also, you must never shop when you are hungry.

You must not only prepare a food list, but you need to make sure that you stick to it while shopping. It is quite easy to cook if you have all the necessary ingredients readily available. Shop for your groceries once a week and if you plan your meals in advance, you will know the groceries you need to buy.

In addition, consider including the following to your shopping list.

- Fish contains good amounts of vitamin D and is rich in proteins and fat. Fish is good for your brain, and since lower calorie intake due to fasting can disrupt your cognition, fish is a great addition to your food cart.

- Cauliflower, Brussels sprouts, broccoli, and other cruciferous veggies. Besides making you feel full (which is how you definitely want to feel if you are going to stay away from eating for 16 long hours!), they can help to prevent constipation during fasting because they are rich in fiber.

- Beans and legumes are low in carbs and can keep your energy up during fasting. Black beans, peas, chickpeas, and lentils can also help in reducing your body weight even when you are not restricting your calorie intake.

- Avocado contains high calories, but the monounsaturated fat in it can keep you full for a long time.

- Whole grains may sound out of place when trying to lose weight because they contain carbs. But they are also rich in protein and fiber. When you eat whole grains instead of refined grains, you are helping to improve your metabolism. So, go for whole grains such as millet, brown rice, oatmeal, spelt, farro, amaranth, whole-wheat bread, and bulgur. As much as possible, limit refined grains such as white flour, white bread, white rice, and degermed cornflower.

- Probiotic-rich foods such as kombucha, kefir, tempeh, and miso are excellent for your gut health.

Chapter 5: 21 days meal plan(with recipe details)

Day 1:

Breakfast

Choco Chip Whey Waffles

Prep time: 10 minutes

Cook time: 6 minutes

Serves: 2

Ingredients:

- 2-tbsp organic coconut oil

- 2-tbsp coconut sugar

- 4-tbsp chocolate whey protein powder

- 1/3 cup almond flour

- A pinch of salt

- ½-tsp baking powder

- ½-cup almond milk

- 2-pcs eggs

Directions:

1. Mix all the ingredients in the blender to obtain a homogenous paste.

2. Preheat your waffle iron. Pour the waffle dough in the iron and cook each waffle for 3 minutes.

Nutritional Value per Serving:

Calories: 423

Fat: 32.8g

Carbs 8.3 g

Protein: 26.5g

Lunch

Flaky Fillets with Garden Greens

Prep Time: 25 minutes

Cook time: 30 minutes

Serves: 4

Ingredients:

- 1-lb broccoli, chopped into cubes and seasoned with a dash of salt and pepper

- 2-tbsp coconut oil

- 7-pcs scallions

- 2-tbsp small capers

- 1-tbsp sesame oil or olive oil

- 1½-lbs. white fish, sliced into 4 fillets

- 1-tbsp dried parsley

- 1¼-cups whipping cream, gluten-free and sugar-free

- 1-tbsp mustard, sugar-free

- 1-tsp of salt

- ¼-tsp ground black pepper

- 1/3 cup olive oil

- 5-oz.leafy greens

Directions:

1. Sauté the seasoned broccoli with sesame oil in a pan, and add the scallions and capers. Add the fish in the middle of the sautéed greens. Simmer for 15 minutes.

2. Meanwhile, mix the parsley with the whipping cream and mustard. Pour it over the cooked fish and vegetables. Drizzle with a little bit of coconut oil.

3. Return the saucepan on medium heat and cook for an extra 10 minutes.

Nutritional Value per Serving:

Calories: 395

Fat: 33g

Carbs 8.7 g

Protein: 19.8g

Dinner

Pizza Pie with Cheesy Cauliflower Crust

Prep time: 5 minutes

Cook time: 30 minutes

Serves: 2

Ingredients:

- ½-head cauliflower, rinsed, riced, cooked for 5 minutes in boiling water, and drained

- 2-pcs eggs, whisked

- 1/3 parmesan cheese

- ½-cup cherry tomatoes, washed and halved

- 2-tbsp organic hempseed oil

- 1-tsp balsamic vinegar

- 1-mozzarella cheese ball, crumbled

- ¼-cup basil leaves

Directions:

1. Spin the cooked cauliflower in a dishtowel to let out as much liquid as possible. (The goal is to obtain a flour texture.) Add the eggs and cheese. Mix well.

2. Spread to a disk the cauliflower dough on a baking pan lined with parchment paper. Bake for 15 minutes at 400°F in your preheated oven.

3. Meanwhile, mix the tomatoes with hempseed oil and balsamic vinegar. Season the mixture with salt and pepper.

4. Remove the pizza dough from the oven. Add the tomato mixture and sprinkle over with mozzarella. Return the pan in the oven and bake further for 15 minutes.

5. Serve hot and garnish with fresh basil leaves.

Nutritional Value per Serving:

Calories: 384

Fat: 32.1g

Carbs 5.5 g

Protein: 19.9g

Day 2:

Breakfast

Coco Cinnamon-Packed Pancakes

Prep time: 30 minutes

Cook time: 5 minutes

Serves: 2

Ingredients:

- 2-pcs eggs

- 2½-tbsp organic coconut flour

- ¼-cup milk substitute with hydrogenated vegetable oil

- 1-tbsp baking soda

- ½-tbsp cinnamon

- ½-tbsp baobab powder

- 2-tbsp organic coconut flower syrup

Directions:

1. In a salad bowl, mix the coconut flour, baobab powder, cinnamon, and baking soda.

2. Add the beaten eggs, the almond milk, and the coconut syrup. Let the dough rest for 30 minutes.

3. Cook the pancakes in a hot pan with coconut oil.

4. Dress the pancakes with raspberries/blueberries or almonds.

Nutritional Value per Serving:

Calories: 392

Fat: 32.5g

Carbs: 11.3 g

Protein 20 g

Lunch

Beef Broccoli with Sesame Sauce

Prep time: 10 minutes

Cook time: 45 minutes

Serves: 4

Ingredients:

- 2-tbsp coconut oil

- 1-tsp arrowroot powder

- 1-tbsp sesame oil

- 1-tbsp red fish sauce

- ½-tsp light sea salt

- ¼-tsp black pepper

- ¼-tsp baking powder

- 1-lb. beef, sliced into ¼-inch thick chunks

- 2-tsp sesame oil or olive oil

- 1-head broccoli, diced

- 2-tbsp coconut oil

- 2-cloves garlic, minced

- 2-ginger, finely chopped

- A pinch of salt and pepper

Directions:

1. Mix the first seven ingredients in a bowl to make the sesame sauce. Set aside.

2. Fry the meat with sesame oil for 15 minutes until browned.

3. In a saucepan with water, add the broccoli, oil, garlic, and ginger. Season it with a pinch of salt and pepper. Add and spread the fried beef with the broccoli. Cover and cook for 20 minutes. Pour the sauce and cook for 10 more minutes.

Nutritional Value per Serving:

Calories: 375

Fat: 31g

Carbs: 5.4 g

Protein: 19.5g

Dinner

Roasted Rib-eye Skillet Steak

Prep time: 5 minutes

Cook time: 15 minutes

Serves: 2

Ingredients:

- 1-16oz rib-eye steak
- 2-tbsp duck fat or peanut oil, divided
- A dash of salt and pepper
- 1-tbsp butter
- ½-tsp thyme, chopped

Directions:

1. Preheat your oven to 400°F. Place a cast iron skillet inside.
2. Season the rib-eye steak with oil, salt, and pepper.
3. Take the preheated skillet out from the oven and place over the stove, set in medium heat. Pour oil, and add the steak. Sear for 2 minutes on both sides.
4. Return the skillet with the steak in the oven. Roast for 6 minutes.

5. Remove the skillet and place over the stove, set in low heat. Add the butter and thyme in the skillet. Baste the steak for about 4 minutes.

Nutritional Value per Serving:

Calories: 722

Fat: 60.2g

Carbs: 1 g

Protein: 45g

Day 3:

Breakfast

Magdalena Muffins with Tart Tomatoes

Prep time: 10 minutes

Cook time: 20 minutes

Serves: 2

Ingredients:

- 2½-tbsp whole-wheat flour

- 2½-tbsp almond flour

- 1-tbsp yeast or baking soda

- A dash of salt, pepper, and paprika

- 2-pcs eggs

- 1-tbsp organic cashew nuts

- 1-tbsp hemp oil

- 2½-tbsp soymilk

- 1/3 cup feta cheese, diced

- 11/3-cup dried tomatoes, without oil and sliced into small pieces

Directions:

1. Mix the wheat flour, almond flour, yeast, and spices.

2. Then add eggs, cashews, oil, and soymilk.

3. Mix well to obtain a smooth paste. Add the feta and tomatoes.

4. Mix well and pour the dough into muffin pans previously greased with coconut oil.

5. Bake for 20 minutes at 350°F.

Nutritional Value per Serving:

Calories: 405

Fat: 33.3g

Carbs: 11 g

Protein: 20.3g

Lunch

Aubergine À la Lasagna

Prep Time: 20 minutes

Cook time: 30 minutes

Serves: 2

Ingredients:

- 2-pcs large eggplants, sliced and drained from excess liquid with a paper towel

- A pinch of sea salt

- 2-cups part-skim ricotta cheese

- ½-cup parmesan cheese, freshly grated

- 1-pc egg, whisked

- 4-cups homemade tomato sauce, sugar-free

- 2-tbsp part-skim mozzarella cheese, shredded

- 2-tbsp cheddar cheese, grated

- 2-tbsp parsley, chopped

Directions:

1. Preheat your oven to 375°F. Meanwhile, season the eggplant slices with salt. Grill the eggplant slices for 3 minutes on each side.

2. Combine the ricotta, parmesan, and egg in a large bowl. Set aside.

3. Spread half of the tomato sauce in a saucepan. Layer half of the eggplant slices, and top with half of the cheddar and mozzarella. Pour half of the ricotta mixture over the layer, or just enough to coat it.

4. Cover the saucepan and insert into your preheated oven. Bake for 25 minutes. Set to cool for 10 minutes.

5. Repeat the process for the second lasagna set. To serve, garnish your lasagna with chopped parsley

Nutritional Value per Serving:

Calories: 346

Fat: 27g

Carbs: 7.9 g

Protein: 21.4g

Dinner

Charred Chicken with Squash Seed Sauce

Prep time: 15 minutes

Cook time: 20 minutes

Serves: 1

Ingredients:

For the Sauce:

- 2-tbsp white almond puree
- 2-cloves of garlic, finely chopped (divided, for the sauce and chicken marinade)
- ½-tbsp squash seeds
- 1-tbsp barley
- 1-pc fresh basil

For the Marinade:

- 2-branches rosemary, finely chopped
- 1-pc red chili, finely chopped
- 1-pc lemon (keep the zest)
- Pinch of salt and ground black pepper
- 1-tbsp olive oil
- 1-cup chicken breasts, cubed

- 5-bulbs small onions, sliced in quarters

- 5-pcs cherry tomatoes

Directions:

1. Combine and mix all the sauce ingredients in a bowl. Set aside.

2. Mix all the marinade ingredients and let stand for 10 minutes. Thread alternately the onions, meat, and tomatoes into the skewers and grill over coal fire for 10 minutes on each side. Serve the chicken kebabs with the squash seed sauce.

Nutritional Value per Serving:

Calories: 428

Fat: 35.6g

Carbs: 16.9 g

Protein: 21g

Day 4:

Breakfast

Spinach Shoots Mediterranean Medley

Prep time: 10 minutes

Cook time: 1 minute

Serves: 2

Ingredients:

- ½-cup spinach shoots

- 2-tbsp quinoa

- ¼-cup avocado, sliced

- 1-tbsp fresh goat cheese

- 1-tsp agave syrup, gluten-free

- ¼-cup dried blackberries

- 1-pc fig

- 1-tsp pumpkin seeds puree

Directions:

1. Arrange the spinach shoots, cooked quinoa, and avocado on a large plate.

2. Mix the goat cheese, agave syrup, and dried blackberries.

3. Make 4 small cuts in the fig so that you can open it and insert the goat cheese mixture.

4. Spread your fig on the spinach shoots. Sprinkle over with pumpkin seed puree.

Nutritional Value per Serving:

Calories: 308

Fat: 26g

Carbs: 9.7 g

Protein: 15.4g

Lunch

Milano Meatballs with Tangy Tomato

Prep Time: 25 minutes

Cook time: 30 minutes

Serves: 3

Ingredients:

For the Meatballs:

- 1-lb extra-lean ground beef

- 1-pc egg, whisked

- 10-pcs sun-dried tomatoes, chopped

- ½-cup ricotta cheese

- 1-cup Parmigiano-Reggiano cheese or parmesan cheese, freshly grated

- A pinch of salt and freshly ground black pepper

For the Tomato Sauce:

- 1-bulb onion, finely chopped

- ¼-cup extra-virgin olive oil

- 2-lbs. tomato puree, gluten-free

- A pinch of salt and freshly ground black pepper

Directions:

1. Combine all the meatball ingredients in a mixing bowl. Mix well until fully combined. Form balls from the mixture, and pat them down for even cooking.

2. Sauté the onions with olive oil in a skillet until they are translucent. Add the tomato puree and bring to a boil. Add the remaining ingredients and the meatballs. Cook for 30 minutes on medium heat.

Nutritional Value per Serving:

Calories: 396

Fat: 32.6g

Carbs: 8.2 g

Protein: 20.9g

Dinner

Therapeutic Turmeric & Shirataki Soup

Prep time: 10 minutes

Cook time: 32 minutes

Serves: 1

Ingredients:

- 1-tbsp turmeric powder

- 1-serving chicken-vegetable broth soup

- 3-pcs carrots, sliced into small pieces

- 3-slices ginger

- 1-pack (5-oz.) konjac shirataki noodles

- ¼-lb. chicken breast, sliced into strips

Directions:

1. Simmer all the ingredients over low heat for 30 minutes.

2. Rinse the konjac noodles thoroughly under cold water.

3. Add the noodles to the broth and heat for 2 minutes.

Nutritional Value per Serving:

Calories: 415

Fat: 34.6g

Carbs: 10.1 g

Protein: 21.6g

Day 5:

Breakfast

Romantic Raspberry Power Pancake

Prep time: 5 minutes

Cook time: 10 minutes

Serves: 3

Ingredients:

- 2-tbsp raspberries, crushed

- 2-tsp almond flour

- 1-tbsp yeast or baking soda

- 1-tbsp vegan protein powder

- 2-tbsp soymilk

- 1-tbsp coconut oil

Directions:

1. Mix the crushed raspberries and dry ingredients.

2. Pour the milk and mix well to obtain a homogenous mixture.

3. Cook the pancakes for 2 minutes on each side using a little coconut oil in a pan. Flip the pancake when small bubbles appear.

4. Dress with almonds or nuts.

Nutritional Value per Serving:

Calories: 323

Fat: 25.3g

Carbs: 12 g

Protein: 15.7g

Lunch

Chicken Curry Masala Mix

Prep Time: 10 minutes

Cook time: 35 minutes

Serves: 3

Ingredients:

- 2-tbsp sesame oil (divided)

- 2-tbsp ginger, diced

- 1½-lbs chicken thighs, boneless, skinless, and diced

- 1-cup tomatoes, chopped

- ¼-cup coriander, chopped

- 2-tsp turmeric

- 1-tsp cumin

- 1-tsp cayenne

- 2-tbsp lemon juice

- Cilantro or mint leaves for garnish

Directions:

1. Sauté the ginger and jalapeno pepper with half of the sesame oil in a saucepan. Add the. Stir in the chicken, tomatoes, and

coriander. Add the spices, the remaining sesame oil, lemon juice and half a cup of water.

2. Cover the saucepan, and cook for 30 minutes.

3. To serve, pour everything in a deep salad bowl, and garnish with cilantro or mint leaves.

Nutritional Value per Serving:

Calories: 377

Fat: 29.3g

Carbs: 6.8 g

Protein: 23.4g

Dinner

Fresh Fettuccine with Pumpkin Pesto

Prep Time: 15 minutes

Cook time: 2 minutes

Serves: 3

Ingredients:

For the Pesto Sauce:

- 1-tbsp olive oil

- 1-tbsp pumpkin seed oil

- ½-tsp pumpkin seeds

- ¼-cup barley

- 1-tbsp lemon juice

- A pinch salt

For the Pasta:

- 1¾-cup zucchini, washed, peeled, and cut into thin noodle strips

- ½-cup cherry tomatoes, washed and cut in half

- 1¼-cup low carb fettuccine

- 1-pc mozzarella cheeseball

- A pinch of pepper

Directions:

1. Combine and mix all the sauce ingredients with 2-tbsp water in a bowl. Set aside.

2. Boil the fettuccine for 1 minute and add the zucchini. Boil further for another minute, and drain.

3. Toss the pasta with the pesto sauce. Season the dish with a pinch of pepper and garnish with tomatoes and mozzarella.

Nutritional Value per Serving:

Calories: 417

Fat: 34.7g

Carbs: 10.5 g

Protein: 20.9g

Day 6:

Breakfast

Mayonnaise Mixed with Energy Egg

Prep time: 2 minutes

Cook time: 5 minutes

Serves: 1

Ingredients:

- 2-tbsp organic mayonnaise, gluten-free

- 1-pc large egg

- 1-tbsp butter

Directions:

1. Mix the mayonnaise and egg in a medium-sized bowl until fully combined.

2. Melt the butter in a non-stick skillet. Pour the egg mixture, and cook until set. Scrape the egg and all remaining fat onto a serving plate. Serve immediately.

Nutritional Value per Serving:

Calories: 295

Fat: 22.7g

Carbs: 3.8 g

Protein: 18.8g

Lunch

Crispy Chicken Packed in Pandan

Prep Time: 30 minutes

Cook time: 18 minutes

Serves: 4

Ingredients:

- 4-pcs (½-lb.) chicken thigh
- 1-tbsp shallot
- 1-pc lemon
- 1-tsp of fennel seeds
- 1-tsp of turmeric powder
- 1-tsp of chili powder
- 1-tbsp of oyster sauce, gluten-free
- A pinch of salt
- A pinch of sugar
- A handful of pandan leaves

Directions:

1. Preheat your air fryer to 350°F for about 5 minutes.

2. Marinate the chicken with all the ingredients. Set aside for 30 minutes.

3. Wrap each chicken meat with the pandan leaves.

4. Arrange the wrapped chicken in the air fryer basket and lock the lid

5. Set to cook for 18 minutes at 375°F.

Nutritional Value per Serving:

Calories: 382

Fat: 32.5g

Protein: 17.8g

Carbs: 7.7 g

Dinner

Cheddar Chicken Casserole

Prep Time: 10 minutes

Cook time: 30 minutes

Serves: 6

Ingredients:

- 20-oz. chicken breasts
- 2-tbsp olive oil, divided
- 2-cups broccoli, steamed
- ½-cup sour cream
- ½-cup heavy cream
- 1-oz. pork rinds, crushed
- A dash of salt and pepper
- ½-tsp paprika
- 1-tsp oregano
- 1-cup cheddar cheese, grated

Directions:

1. Preheat your oven to 450°F.

2. Sear the chicken with a tablespoon of olive oil in a pan until it cooks all the way through. Shred the meat in the pan. Add the remaining oil, broccoli, and sour cream.

3. Place and spread evenly the mixture in an 8" x11" pan. Press firmly and drizzle with heavy cream. Add all the remaining seasonings and top the casserole with the cheese. Place the pan in the oven and bake for 25 minutes until the edges turn brown and start bubbling.

Nutritional Value per Serving:

Calories: 405

Fat: 33.8g

Protein: 22.7g

Carbs: 3.6 g

Day 7:

Breakfast

Avocados Toasted Tartiné

Prep time: 10 minutes

Cook time: 5 minutes

Serves: 2

Ingredients:

- 2-slices bread, gluten-free
- ½-pc small avocado, thinly sliced
- 1-tbsp fresh cheese
- 1-tsp lemon juice
- A dash of salt and pepper
- 1-tsp chia seeds for garnish (optional)

Directions:

1. Toast lightly the bread slices.

2. Carefully arrange the avocado slices on each bread slice. Drizzle with the lemon juice. Spread the fresh cheese. Sprinkle with a dash of salt and pepper. Top with garnish.

Nutritional Value per Serving:

Calories: 268

Fat: 22.4g

Protein: 13.5g

Carbs: 8.9 g

Lunch

Stuffed Straw Mushroom Mobcap

Prep Time: 15 minutes

Cook time: 5 minutes

Serves: 1

Ingredients:

- 1-cup fresh spinach, washed, bathed in ice, and drained

- 1-cup straw mushrooms or Chinese mushroom, washed and stems removed

- 1-tbsp coconut oil

- 1-bulb onion, finely chopped

- 1-clove garlic, minced

- A dash of salt and pepper

- A pinch of nutmeg

- ¼-cup quinoa, cooked

- 3.5-oz. cottage cheese

Directions:

1. Spread the spinach leaves over the food film while rolling them.

2. Fry the mushrooms with coconut oil in a saucepan before adding onion and garlic. Season the mushrooms with salt, pepper, and nutmeg. Set aside.

3. Combine the cooked quinoa with the cottage cheese. Spread the mixture evenly on the spinach leaves then roll into a pudding with the help of the food film.

4. Stuff the mushroom heads with the spinach pudding, and place them in the fridge.

5. Just before serving, slice the mushroom head with a sharp knife and pass quickly to the pan to heat.

Nutritional Value per Serving:

Calories: 401

Fat: 34.7g

Protein: 17.2g

Carbs: 16.9 g

Dinner

Zesty Zucchini Pseudo Pasta & Sweet Spanish Onions Overload

Prep Time: 10 minutes

Cook time: 20 minutes

Serves: 2

Ingredients:

- 2-tbsp of vegetable oil

- 2-pcs yellow onions or Spanish onions

- 1-tbsp soy sauce, low-sodium

- 2-tbsp teriyaki sauce, low-sodium

- 1-tbsp sesame seeds

- 4-pcs small zucchinis, sliced into spaghetti strips using a spiral cutter

Directions:

1. Add the vegetable oil, onions, and soy sauce to a saucepan placed over medium heat. Stir in the teriyaki sauce and sesame seeds. Mix well until fully combined.

2. Cook for 10 minutes, stirring frequently until the vegetables turn brown.

3. Add the zucchini pasta and cook for 3 minutes.

4. To serve, transfer the pasta in a serving dish and garnish with chopped parsley.

Nutritional Value per Serving:

Calories: 319

Fat: 25.9g

Protein: 18.1g

Carbs: 6.6 g

Day 8:

Breakfast

Fish Fillet & Perky Potato Cheese Combo

Prep time: 15 minutes

Cook time: 10 minutes

Serves: 2

Ingredients:

- 1-tbsp olive oil

- 1-pc large potato, cooked and thinly sliced

- ¼-cup lean white cheese

- ½-tsp herbs of your choice

- 3.5-oz. herring fillet, steamed and sliced in half

- ½-tsp flaxseed oil or coconut oil

- A dash of salt and pepper

Directions:

1. Heat a non-stick pan with olive oil. Add the potato slices and cook until browned.

2. Season the white cheese with salt, pepper, and herbs of your choice.

3. Arrange the potatoes equally between two plates. Top with the cheese and herring fillets. Garnish with a drizzle of flaxseed oil.

Nutritional Value per Serving:

Calories: 298

Fat: 24.9g

Protein: 14.2g

Carbs: 6.5 g

Lunch

Tasty Tofu Carrots &Cauliflower Cereal

Prep Time: 20 minutes

Cook time: 20 minutes

Serves: 1

Ingredients:

For the Tofu-Carrots Mix:

- ½-block extra firm tofu, crumbled
- 2-tbsp reduced sodium soy sauce, gluten-free
- ½-cup onion, diced
- 1-cup carrot, diced
- 1-tsp turmeric

For the Cauliflower Cereal:

- 3-cups riced cauliflower
- 2-tbsp reduced sodium soy sauce, gluten-free
- 1½-tsp toasted sesame oil
- 1-tbsp rice vinegar
- 1-tbsp ginger, minced
- ½-cup broccoli, finely chopped

279

- 2-cloves garlic, minced

- ½-cup frozen peas

Directions:

1. Toss the tofu with the rest of the tofu-carrots mix ingredients. Place the mixture in your air fryer basket. Lock the lid, and set to cook for 10 minutes at 370°F.

2. Meanwhile, toss together all of the cauliflower cereal ingredients. Add this mixture to the air fryer pan. Lock the lid, and set to cook for another 10 minutes at 375°F.

Nutritional Value per Serving:

Calories: 390

Fat: 32.6g

Protein: 19.5g

Carbs: 17.4 g

Dinner

Soba & Spinach Sprouts

Prep Time: 15 minutes

Cook time: 0 minutes

Serves: 2

Ingredients:

- 3-pcs mushrooms, sliced into quarters

- 1/3 cup smoked tofu, sliced into squares

- 1-tbsp coconut oil

- ½-pc green pepper, sliced into strips

- 3-tbsp cashew nuts

- ½- clove garlic

- ½-pc lime, juice

- A dash of salt and pepper

- ¼-cup water (more, as needed)

- ¼-cup soba noodles, cooked according to package instructions

- 11/3-cup spinach sprouts

- 1-tbsp coconut shavings for garnish

Directions:

1. Fry the mushrooms and tofu with coconut oil in a frying pan until they turn brown. Add the pepper. Set aside.

2. For the sauce, mix cashews with garlic, lime juice, salt, pepper, and a little water.

3. Divide the noodles between two bowls and top with spinach sprouts. Arrange the remaining vegetables on top. Garnish with coconut shavings or avocado slices, sesame seeds, and a slice of lime.

4. To serve, pour over the sauce on each arranged bowl.

Nutritional Value per Serving:

Calories: 355

Fat: 29.6g

Protein: 17.8g

Carbs: 8.3 g

Day 9:

Breakfast

Cream Cheese Protein Pancake

Prep time: 10 minutes

Cook time: 12 minutes

Serves: 2

Ingredients:

- 2-pcs eggs

- 2-oz cream cheese

- 1-packet sweetener

- ½-tsp cinnamon

- 1-tbsp butter

Directions:

1. Combine all the ingredients except the butter in a blender. Blend until smooth. Let the batter stand for 2 minutes to allow the bubbles to settle.

2. Grease slightly a hot pan with ¼-tbsp butter. Pour ¼-batter into the pan. Cook for about 2 minutes until turning golden. Flip the pancake and cook for 1 minute on its other side.

3. Repeat the same cooking procedure with the remaining batter. Serve with fresh berries of choice and sugar-free syrup.

Nutritional Value per Serving:

Calories: 340

Fat: 28.1g

Protein: 16.2g

Carbs: 8.1 g

Lunch

Prawn Pasta

Prep Time: 10 minutes

Cook time: 12 minutes

Serves: 3

Ingredients:

- 1-tsp sesame seeds

- 1-pc lime

- ½-pc green pepper, thinly sliced

- 2 tbsp coconut flour

- 2-tbsp sesame oil

- 1-tbsp soy sauce, gluten-free

- 2-heads small cabbages

- 6-bulbs small onions, chopped

- 1-cup prawns, steamed

- 3-cups low-carb pasta, rinsed, drained, and cooked for 2 minutes in boiling water

- 8-pcs small radishes, sliced into 4-pieces for garnish

- ½-pc avocado, sliced for garnish

Directions:

1. Combine the first six ingredients in a bowl to make the pasta sauce. Set aside.

2. Cook the cabbage for 10 minutes in a pan with a little water and soy sauce. Add the onions and prawns. Cook for 2 minutes.

3. Arrange the pasta in a plate, topped with the prawn mixture, pasta sauce, and the garnishing.

Nutritional Value per Serving:

Calories: 393

Fat: 32.8g

Protein: 19.7g

Carbs: 14.9 g

Dinner

Chickpeas & Carrot Consommé

Prep Time: 10 minutes

Cook time: 20 minutes

Serves: 2

Ingredients:

- ¼-lb. chickpeas, cooked
- 1-tbsp coconut oil
- 1-clove garlic, minced
- 1-piece ginger, minced
- 1-bulb small onion, finely chopped
- ½-lb. carrots, sliced into small pieces
- 1¼-cup vegetable broth
- A dash of salt and pepper
- ½-cup coconut milk
- 1-tbsp coconut shaving

Directions:

1. Arrange the chickpeas on a plate lined with parchment paper. Sprinkle with salt, curry, and paprika. Spread the spices well and bake for 15 minutes at 350°F.

2. Melt the coconut oil in a saucepan and brown the garlic, ginger, and onion. Add the carrots. Deglaze with vegetable broth and simmer for 15 minutes over medium heat until the carrots cook through.

3. Season to taste with salt, pepper, curry, and paprika. Pour the coconut milk.

4. Mix the soup and garnish with chickpeas and coconut shavings.

Nutritional Value per Serving:

Calories: 460

Fat: 38.2g

Protein: 23.3g

Carbs: 10.1 g

Day 10:

Breakfast

Veggie Variety with Peanut Paste

Prep time: 15 minutes

Cook time: 15 minutes

Serves: 1

Ingredients:

- 1-bulb small onion, thinly sliced

- ¾-cup broccoli, sliced into quarters

- 1-pc small carrot, sliced into quarters

- ½-pc green pepper, thinly sliced

- 5-pcs mushrooms, sliced into quarters

- A dash of salt, pepper, and powdered chili

- 2-tbsp peanut butter, dairy-free

- 2-tbsp. soy sauce, gluten-free

- 1-tbsp agave syrup (or honey), gluten-free

- ¼-cup red cabbage, thinly sliced

Directions:

1. Pour a little water in a heated skillet and cook the onions until they are transparent. Add the broccoli, carrot, pepper, and mushrooms. Cook for 10 minutes until tender. (Add a little water if the pan is too dry). Season the veggies with a dash of salt, pepper, and chili.

2. For the sauce, mix the peanut butter with the soy sauce, agave syrup, and 3 tbsp water.

3. To serve, incorporate the red cabbage. Garnish the dish with the sauce.

Nutritional Value per Serving:

Calories: 349

Fat: 28.7g

Protein: 18.4g

Carbs: 10.8 g

Lunch

Stuffed Spaghetti Squash

Prep Time: 30 minutes

Cook time: 30 minutes

Serves: 2

Ingredients:

- 1-pc spaghetti squash, halved and pitted
- 1-tsp olive oil
- ½-cup bacon strips, grilled
- 3-cups ground beef
- 1-pc green pepper, thinly sliced
- ½-bulb onion, sliced into cubes
- 1-tsp garlic powder
- 1-tsp paprika
- A pinch of salt and pepper
- 1-cup cheddar cheese, grated

Directions:

1. Rub the squash halves with oil, and bake for 30 minutes at 350°F.

2. Meanwhile, roast the bacon in a saucepan placed over high heat. Stir in the onion and pepper. Add the beef and spices. Season the mixture with salt and pepper, and cook for 15 minutes, stirring regularly. Set aside.

3. Remove the flesh of the cooked squash by scratching with a fork. Mix the flesh with the meat mixture. Add the cheese, and put the mixture in the frayed squash.

4. Return the stuffed squash to the hot oven, and bake for 10 minutes.

Nutritional Value per Serving:

Calories: 404

Fat: 33.2g

Protein: 20.3g

Carbs: 7 g

Dinner

Chicken Cauliflower Curry

Prep Time: 15 minutes

Cook time: 30 minutes

Serves: 2

Ingredients

- 1-cup vegetable broth
- 1-tbsp curry paste
- ½-cup light coconut milk
- ½-lb chicken breast, cooked and sliced into small pieces
- 1-pc potato, diced
- 1-clove garlic, minced
- ½-bulb onion, finely chopped
- 1-cup cauliflower, diced
- 1/3-cup fresh peas
- Salt and pepper
- ¼-cup goji berries

Directions:

1. Heat the vegetable broth in a wok for 5 minutes. Add the curry paste, coconut milk, meat, potato, garlic, and onion. Cook for 15 minutes.

2. Add the vegetables and cook further for 10 minutes until they are tender. Season the curry with a dash of salt and pepper.

3. To serve, garnish with goji berries.

Nutritional Value per Serving:

Calories: 334

Fat: 27g

Protein: 18.7g

Carbs: 8.4 g

Day 11:

Breakfast

Avocado Aliment with Egg Element

Prep time: 8 minutes

Cook time: 20 minutes

Serves: 2

Ingredients:

- 1-pc egg, whisked
- 1-pc avocado, halved, pitted, and removed slightly with flesh
- A dash of sea salt and pepper
- 1-tbsp parsley, chopped
- 1-tsp cayenne pepper

Directions:

1. Preheat your oven to 375°F.
2. Pour the egg gently into each halved avocado. Remove the excess liquid.
3. Place the stuffed avocado in a baking tray. Bake for 20 minutes.
4. Season the preparation with sea salt, parsley, and cayenne pepper.

Nutritional Value per Serving:

Calories: 275

Fat: 23.8g

Protein: 11.8g

Carbs: 10.7 g

Lunch

Steamed Salmon & Salad Bento Box

Prep Time: 10 minutes

Cook time: 0 minutes

Serves: 2

Ingredients:

- 2-pcs salad heads

- 1-cup carrot, grated

- ¼-cup cucumber, sliced

- 1-pc green pepper, thinly sliced

- 4-cups marinara pasta, rinsed, drained, and cooked for 2 minutes in boiling water

- ½-lb. salmon, steamed

- 2-pcs lemons

- 2-pcs eggs, boiled and sliced

- 1-tsp chia seeds

- 4-tbsp yogurt, sugar-free

- 1-tsp turmeric powder

- ½-pc lemon, zest

- 2-tbsp mint, minced

- A pinch of pepper

Directions:

1. Divide equally the first eight ingredients between two bento boxes. Sprinkle the arrangements with chia seeds.

2. Mix the rest of the ingredients to make the sauce. Pack the sauce separately.

Nutritional Value per Serving:

Calories: 391

Fat: 30.4g

Protein: 24.9g

Carbs: 11.8 g

Dinner

Cheesy Cauliflower Mac Munchies

Prep Time: 20 minutes

Cook time: 15 minutes

Serves: 2

Ingredients:

- 1-pc medium cauliflower, riced
- 3-tbsp + ½-tsp avocado oil, divided
- A pinch of sea salt
- A pinch of black pepper
- 1-cup cheddar cheese, shredded
- ¼-cup cream, gluten-free
- ¼-cup almond milk, unsweetened

Directions:

1. Preheat your air fryer to 400°F. Spray the pan with oil.
2. Place the riced cauliflower in the pan and drizzle with the avocado oil. Toss well and season with a pinch each of salt and pepper. Set aside.
3. Heat the cheese, cream, and milk with a little bit of avocado oil in a pot.

4. Pour the cheese mixture over the seasoned cauliflower. Lock the lid of the air fryer and set to cook for 14 minutes.

Nutritional Value per Serving:

Calories: 352

Fat: 27.8g

Protein: 20.9g

Carbs: 8.9 g

Day 12:

Breakfast

Pumpkin Pancakes

Prep time: 10 minutes

Cook time: 30 minutes

Serves: 3

Ingredients:

- 1-tsp vanilla extract
- 1-cup coconut cream
- 3-pcs eggs
- 2-tbsp egg whites
- ½-cup pumpkin puree
- 5-packs sweetener
- 4-tbsp ground flax seed
- 4-tbsp ground hazelnuts or hazelnut flour
- 1-tsp yeast or baking powder
- 1-tbsp black tea powder
- 1-tbsp. coconut oil for cooking

Directions:

1. Whisk together the first five liquid ingredients for half a minute until they become frothy. Mix the dry ingredients in a separate bowl.

2. Combine both the dry and liquid ingredients to obtain a batter. (Add water, as necessary if the mixture is too thick.)

3. Grease a saucepan with a teaspoon of coconut oil. Ladle in the first pancake.

4. Cover the pan and cook for 3 minutes. Flip and cook the other side.

5. Repeat the cooking process until using up all the batter.

Nutritional Value per Serving:

Calories: 200

Fat: 16.4g

Protein: 11g

Carbs: 5.2 g

Lunch

Smoky Sage Sausage

Prep Time: 5 minutes

Cook time: 8 minutes

Serves: 4

Ingredients:

- 2-tbsp sage, chopped
- 2-packets sweetener
- 1-tsp salt
- 1-tsp maple extract
- 1-lb. ground pork
- ½-tsp black pepper
- ¼-tsp garlic powder
- 1/8-tsp cayenne pepper

Directions:

1. Combine all the ingredients in a large mixing bowl.
2. Form patties from the mixture.
3. Put the patties in a skillet placed over medium heat. Cook for 4 minutes until cooked through. Flip the patties to cook on the other side.

Nutritional Value per Serving:

Calories: 170

Fat: 13.2g

Protein: 8.4g

Carbs: 5.3 g

Dinner

Sugar Snap Pea Pods with Coco Crunch

Prep Time: 5 minutes

Cook time: 10 minutes

Serves: 2

Ingredients:

- 4-tbsp salted butter, gluten-free and dairy-free

- 1-tbsp coconut oil

- ½-cup coconut, unsweetened and shredded

- 1/8-tsp cinnamon

- 1-tbsp rosemary oil

- 9-oz. snap pea pods, trimmed, strings removed, and diced

- A pinch of salt

Directions:

1. In a saucepan, melt the coconut oil with the butter over medium heat. Add the coconut shreds, rosemary oil, and cinnamon. Toss very well until fully incorporated.

2. Add the diced pea pods and mix again. Leave to cook for 8 minutes until the pea pods start to melt.

3. To serve, sprinkle over a pinch of salt.

Nutritional Value per Serving:

Calories: 389

Fat: 31.3g

Protein: 22g

Carbs: 7.2 g

Day 13:

Breakfast

Whole-Wheat Plain Pancakes

Prep time: 5 minutes

Cook time: 12 minutes

Serves: 1

Ingredients:

- 2-pcs eggs

- 4-tbsp whole-wheat flour

- ½-tsp yeast or baking soda

- 1/3-cup sunflower oil

- 1-tbsp coconut oil for cooking

Directions:

1. Mix all the ingredients in a bowl until obtaining a smooth consistency.

2. Pour the coconut oil in a pan placed over medium heat. Cook for 3 minutes until browned. Flip and cook the other side.

3. Serve hot and garnish with fresh fruits of your choice such as blueberries, strawberries or raspberries, nuts, and coconut flakes.

Nutritional Value per Serving:

Calories: 329

Fat: 27.6g

Protein: 16.1g

Carbs: 5.4 g

Lunch

Bunless Bacon Burger

Prep Time: 8 minutes

Cook time: 37 minutes

Serves: 4

Ingredients:

- 1½-lbs. ground beef
- 2-tbsp olive oil
- 2-tbsp bacon bits
- 4-oz. pepper jack cheese
- 1-bulb onion, sliced crosswise
- 8-leaves romaine lettuce
- A dash of salt and pepper

Directions:

1. Form the ground beef into four patties. Cook for 4 minutes with olive oil on a skillet placed over medium heat. Flip the patties to cook the other sides. Set aside.

2. Using the same skillet, stir-fry the bacon bits for 5 minutes until crispy.

3. Use the lettuce leaves as buns. Place each patty on a leaf and top with the bacon bits. Sprinkle a dash of salt and pepper. Top each burger with the cheese to melt.

Nutritional Value per Serving:

Calories: 435

Fat: 36.3g

Protein: 21.7g

Carbs: 6.1 g

Dinner

Spicy & Smoky Spinach-Set Fish Fillets

Prep Time: 15 minutes

Cook time: 10 minutes

Serves: 2

Ingredients:

- 2-pcs halibut meat (11-oz. each), membrane removed and deboned

- 4-cups packed spinach

- Juice of ½-pc lemon

- A pinch of salt and pepper

- A pinch of smoked paprika

- 1-pc sliced lemon

- 1-pc green onions, sliced

- 1-pc red chili, deseeded and thinly sliced

- 1-cup cherry tomatoes, halved

- 2-tbsp avocado oil

Directions:

1. Place the halibut meat over a flat surface. Divide the spinach between them.

311

2. Lay each halibut meat on each pile of spinach. Squeeze the lemon over each part and season with smoked paprika.

3. Top each fish meat with lemon slices, green onions, chili, and the cherry tomatoes. Pour 1-tbsp of avocado oil over each fish portion.

4. Wrap around each fish meat tightly with foil; arrange them in a baking pan. Cook for 10 mins until the fish turns golden and flaky when forked.

Nutritional Value per Serving:

Calories: 248

Fat: 18.8g

Protein: 15.3g

Carbs: 13.2 g

Day 14:

Breakfast

Blueberries Breakfast Bowl

Prep time: 35 minutes

Cook time: 0 minutes

Serves: 1

Ingredients:

- 1-tsp chia seeds

- 1-cup almond milk

- ¼-cup fresh blueberries or fresh fruits

- 1-pack sweetener for taste

Directions:

1. Mix the chia seeds with the almond milk. Stir periodically.

2. Place in the fridge to cool for 30 minutes, and then serve with fresh fruit. Enjoy!

Nutritional Value per Serving:

Calories: 202

Fat: 16.8g

Protein: 10.2g

Carbs: 9.8 g

Lunch

Baked Broccoli in Olive Oil

Prep Time: 5 minutes

Cook time: 25 minutes

Serves: 3

Ingredients:

- 1½-lbs broccoli florets
- ¼-cup olive oil
- 3-tsps garlic, minced
- 2-tbsp fresh basil, chopped
- ½-tsp red chili flakes
- ¾-tsp kosher salt
- Zest of ½-pc lemon
- Juice of ½-pc lemon
- 1/3cup parmesan cheese

Directions:

1. Preheat your oven to 425°F.

2. Arrange the broccoli florets in a baking sheet lined with parchment paper.

3. Season the broccoli with olive oil, chopped fresh basil, minced garlic, kosher salt, red chili flakes, zest and juice of half a lemon each.

4. Sprinkle parmesan cheese over the broccoli. Place the sheet in the oven to bake for about 25 minutes.

Nutritional Value per Serving:

Calories: 484

Fat: 39.2g

Protein: 26.7g

Carbs: 21.6 g

Dinner

Spicy Shrimps & Sweet Shishito

Prep Time: 15 minutes

Cook time: 15 minutes

Serves: 2

Ingredients:

- 2-tbsp canola oil

- A pinch of sea salt

- 1-clove garlic, crushed and finely chopped

- 1-pc red chili pepper, seeded and finely chopped

- 5-oz. whole shishito peppers

- 10-oz. shrimps, jumbo size

- 1-tsp sesame oil

- 2-tbsp low-sodium light soy sauce

- Juice of 1-pc lime

Directions:

1. Preheat your air fryer to 350°F for about 5 minutes. Spray your air fryer pan with canola oil.

2. Add the salt, garlic, and red chili pepper. Mix well until fully combined.

3. Add the shishito peppers; mix thoroughly again. Add the shrimps and drizzle with sesame oil.

4. Place the pan in your air fryer and lock the lid. Cook for about 10 minutes at 400°F

5. Divide the dish equally between three serving bowls. To serve, season each bowl with lime juice and soy sauce.

Nutritional Value per Serving:

Calories: 370

Fat: 28.9g

Protein: 23g

Carbs 7.2 g

Day 15:

Breakfast

Feta-Filled Tomato-Topped Oldie Omelet

Prep time: 5 minutes

Cook time: 6 minutes

Serves: 1

Ingredients:

- 1-tbsp coconut oil

- 2-pcs eggs

- 1½-tbsp milk

- A dash of salt and pepper

- ¼-cup tomatoes, sliced into cubes

- 2-tbsp feta cheese, crumbled

Directions:

1. Beat the eggs with the milk, salt, pepper, and the remaining spices.

2. Pour the mixture into a heated pan with coconut oil.

3. Stir in the tomatoes and cheese. Cook for 6 minutes or until the cheese melts.

Nutritional Value per Serving:

Calories: 335

Fat: 28.4g

Protein: 16.2g

Carbs: 4.5 g

Lunch

Chickpeas Carrots Curry

Prep time: 5 minutes

Cook time: 25 minutes

Serves: 1

Ingredients:

- ½-bulb onion, finely chopped

- ½-pc carrot, sliced into cubes

- ½ tsp coconut oil

- ¼-cup chickpeas

- ½-tsp tomato paste

- 3-tbsp light soy cream

- ½-tsp turmeric powder

- 1/8-bunch fresh coriander

- A pinch of salt, pepper, and sweet paprika

Directions:

1. Sauté the onions and carrots for 5 minutes with coconut oil in a skillet.

2. Add the chickpeas, tomato paste, soy cream, turmeric, coriander, and spices. Mix well and cook for 10 minutes.

3. Cook the rice for 10 minutes in boiling water. Serve the konjac rice with the vegetable curry and chickpeas.

Nutritional Value per Serving:

Calories: 380

Fat: 30.9g

Protein: 18g

Carbs: 14.4 g

Dinner

Spaghetti-Styled Zesty Zucchini with Guacamole Garnish

Prep Time: 15 minutes

Cook time: 5 minutes

Serves: 2

Ingredients:

- 2-pcs medium zucchini, cut into spaghetti strips using a spiral cutter

- 1-tbsp sea salt

- 1-pc large avocado, peeled, pitted, and cut into small pieces

- 11/3-cup fresh basil, washed, dried and finely chopped

- 2-tbsp lemon juice

- A dash of salt and black pepper

- 1-tbsp coconut oil

- 7-oz. mushrooms, cleaned and cut into slices

- 1-pc pomegranate, seeds extracted

Directions:

1. Season the zucchini strips with sea salt and set aside.

2. Mix the avocado slices, lemon juice, and a dash of salt and pepper. Set aside.

3. Toss lightly the zucchini in a frying pan placed over medium heat. Fry for 4 to 5 minutes in coconut oil. Add the mushrooms and pomegranate seeds.

4. To serve, place the zucchini spaghetti on a plate with the avocado cream in a separate bowl. Garnish with the basil leaves.

Nutritional Value per Serving:

Calories: 381

Fat: 31.8g

Protein: 19g

Carbs: 14.3 g

Day 17:

Breakfast

Ave Avocado Super Smoothie

Prep time: 10 minutes

Cook time: 1 minute

Serves: 1

Ingredients:

- ½-cup Greek yogurt
- 7-oz. frozen avocados
- ½-cup water
- ½-tsp vanilla powder
- 1-tsp each chia seeds, chocolate chips, and peanut butter for garnish

Directions:

1. Mix all the ingredients. You can also crush them in the blender.
2. Pour the smoothie into a bowl and garnish to your taste with fruits, seeds or nuts.

Nutritional Value per Serving:

Calories: 398

Fat: 33.1g

Protein: 20g

Carbs: 15.5 g

Lunch

Poultry Pâté & Creamy Crackers

Prep time: 15 minutes

Cook time: 35 minutes

Serves: 1

Ingredients:

- 3.5-oz. chicken livers

- 3-tbsp butter, softened

- 1-tsp. Italian seasoning

- A pinch of salt and pepper

- 3-pcs unsalted creamy crackers, gluten-free

Directions:

1. Place all the ingredients in a blender except the crackers. Blend to a smooth paste consistency.

2. Serve with the crackers.

Nutritional Value per Serving:

Calories: 437

Fat: 36.4g

Protein: 21.9g

Carbs: 5.5 g

Dinner

Grain-less Gnocchi in Melted Mozzarella

Prep Time: 10 minutes

Cook time: 15 minutes

Serves: 1

Ingredients:

- 2-cups mozzarella, shredded

- ½-tsp garlic powder

- 1-tsp salt

- 3-pcs large egg yolks, whisked, divided

- ½-cup tomato sauce, gluten-free

Directions:

1. Melt the mozzarella with the garlic powder and salt for 5 minutes in a microwave-safe dish.

2. Pour half of the egg yolks into the mozzarella mixture in a large bowl. Mix until fully combined. Add the remaining egg yolks. Mix thoroughly again until fully incorporated.

3. Divide the mixture into four parts. Roll each part into a long rope over a flat surface. Cut each rope into gnocchi-like pieces, pressing each with a fork.

4. Bring a pan filled with water to a boil. Add the gnocchi dumplings and cook for about 2 minutes.

5. Preheat your air fryer to 350°F. Spray the air fryer pan with cooking oil.

6. Arrange the gnocchi pieces in the air fryer pan. Lock the lid of the air fryer and cook for 10 minutes.

7. To serve, pour the tomato sauce over the gnocchi.

Nutritional Value per Serving:

Calories: 355

Fat: 27.6g

Protein: 22.1g

Carbs: 6.5 g

Day 18:

Breakfast

Hearty Hodgepodge

Prep time: 5 minutes

Cook time: 25 minutes

Serves: 1

Ingredients:

- 1-bulb small onion, diced

- 1-tbsp coconut oil

- 1-tbsp bacon bits

- 1-pc medium zucchini, diced into squares

- 1-tbsp parsley or chives, chopped

- ¼-tsp. of salt

- 1-pc large egg, fried

Directions:

1. Sauté the onion with coconut oil in a pan placed over medium heat. Add the bacon, stirring frequently until both onion and bacon turn slightly brown.

2. Add the zucchini, and cook for 15 minutes. Remove from heat and transfer the preparation in a serving bowl. Sprinkle over the parsley.

3. To serve, top the dish with the fried egg.

Nutritional Value per Serving:

Calories: 290

Fat: 24g

Protein: 14.6g

Carbs: 6.7 g

Lunch

Single Skillet Seafood-Filled Frittata

Prep time: 2 minutes

Cook time: 18 minutes

Serves: 4

Ingredients:

- 1-pc green pepper
- ¼-pc lime, squeezed for juice
- 1-tbsp coconut flour
- 1-tbsp sesame oil
- 1-tbsp soy sauce, gluten-free
- 1-tbsp coconut oil
- 3-bulbs fresh onions, chopped
- ½-clove garlic, minced
- ¼-cup prawns, raw
- 11/3-cup mussels, deshelled
- 2-pcs eggs, whisked

Directions:

1. Preheat your oven to 475°F. Meanwhile, make the sauce by combining the first five ingredients in a mixing bowl. Mix thoroughly until fully combined. Set aside.

2. Melt the coconut oil in a small skillet and fry the onions. Add the garlic, prawns, and mussels. Cook for 10 minutes until the prawns turn pink.

3. Stir in the eggs. Place the skillet in the oven and bake for 5 minutes.

4. Slice the frittata in four slices and serve with the sauce.

Nutritional Value per Serving:

Calories: 459

Fat: 38.2g

Protein: 22.9g

Carbs: 8.7 g

Dinner

Cauliflower Chao Fan Fried with Pork Pastiche

Prep Time: 20 minutes

Cook time: 15 minutes

Serves: 4

Ingredients:

- ½-head medium-sized cauliflower, chopped into small cubes
- 2-pcs eggs
- 2-cloves garlic, chopped
- 2-cups pork belly, cut into thin strips
- 3-pcs green capsicums
- 2-bulbs onions
- 1-tbsp soy sauce, gluten-free
- 1-tsp black sesame seeds
- 1-tbsp spring onion, chopped
- 1-tsp pickled ginger

Directions:

1. Place the chopped cauliflower in your food processor; pulse into smaller granules. Set aside.

2. Whisk the eggs, and swirl in the frying pan. Cook for 3 minutes.

3. Add the pork belly strips and the cauliflower rice. Stir in the onions and soy sauce. Cook for about 10 minutes.

4. To serve, distribute the preparation equally between four serving bowls. Garnish with sesame seeds, spring onions, and pickled ginger.

Nutritional Value per Serving:

Calories: 460

Fat: 35.7g |

Protein: 28.6g

Carbs: 8.3 g

Day 19:

Breakfast

Chocolate Chia Plain Pudding

Prep time: 55 minutes

Cook time: 0 minutes

Serves: 3

Ingredients:

- 3-tbsp chia seeds

- 2-cups water

- ¼-cup whey chocolate protein

- ½-cup Greek yogurt, sugar-free

- ¼-cup linseeds, roasted

- 1-tbsp cocoa powder, unsweetened

- 1-packet sweetener (optional)

Directions:

1. Mix the chia seeds with water and let stand for 20 minutes. Stir occasionally.

2. Once the chia seeds are well inflated, add all the other ingredients and mix again.

3. Place in the fridge for 30 minutes before serving.

Nutritional Value per Serving:

Calories: 370

Fat: 28.7g

Protein: 22.3g

Carbs: 10.8 g

Lunch

Shrimps & Spinach Spaghetti

Prep time: 5 minutes

Cook time: 8 minutes

Serves: 2

Ingredients:

- 8-tbsp vegetable broth

- 1-cup low carb spaghetti, rinsed and drained

- 1-pc leek, cut into strips

- 11/3-cup frozen peas

- 11/3-cup fresh spinach leaves

- ¼-lb. shrimp, pre-cooked

- 1-tbsp lemon zest

- 1-pc green pepper, finely chopped

- 2-pcs basil leaves

- 1-pc lemon

Directions:

1. Pour the vegetable broth in a wok and cook for 5 minutes. Add the leeks, peas, spinach, and shrimp. Cook further for 5 minutes.

338

2. Add the spaghetti, and continue cooking for 2 minutes. Remove quickly from heat and pour into a bowl, mix with lemon zest.

3. Divide the pasta equally between two plates. To serve, garnish with the pepper, basil leaves, and lemon.

Nutritional Value per Serving:

Calories: 425

Fat: 33g

Protein: 25g

Carbs: 15.7 g

Dinner

Philadelphia Potato Praline

Prep time: 30 minutes

Cook time: 0 minutes

Serves: 2

Ingredients:

- 1/3-cup Philadelphia cream cheese

- 1½-cup coconut, unsweetened and shredded

- 1-tbsp butter

- ¼-tsp ground cinnamon

- Sweetener of choice

Directions:

1. Combine all the ingredients except for the ground cinnamon in a bowl. Refrigerate the mixture and allow setting until it hardens.

2. Divide the mixture into 8 portions and roll each portion into potato shapes. Place them on a sheet of parchment paper.

3. Sprinkle all over with the cinnamon and store in the fridge for a week before serving.

Nutritional Value per Serving:

Calories: 180

Fat: 15.3g

Protein: 8.9g

Carbs: 3.2 g

Day 20:

Breakfast

Seasoned Sardines with Sunny Side

Prep time: 5 minutes

Cook time: 10 minutes

Serves: 1

Ingredients:

- 2-oz. sardines in olive oil
- 2-pcs eggs
- ½-cup arugula
- ¼-cup artichoke hearts, diced
- A pinch of salt
- A dash of black pepper

Directions:

1. Preheat your oven to 375°F.

2. Place the sardines in an oven-ready stoneware bowl. Add the eggs on top of the sardines. Top the eggs with the arugula and artichokes. Sprinkle with salt and pepper.

3. Bake for 10 minutes until the eggs cook through.

Nutritional Value per Serving:

Calories: 255

Fat: 21g

Carbs: 4.9 g

Protein: 13.5g

Lunch

Pulled Pepper-Lemon Loins

Prep time: 15 minutes

Cook time: 240-360 minutes

Serves: 4

Ingredients

- ½-stick of butter
- 1-pc large lemon, sliced
- 1-pc green pepper, chopped
- 1-tbsp garlic, minced
- 2-tbsp olive oil
- 1-tbsp salt
- 1-tsp dried thyme
- ½-tbsp Dijon mustard
- 3-lbs. (4-pcs) chicken tenderloins
- 1-cheddar cheese slice, shredded
- 4-leaves romaine lettuce

Directions:

1. Combine the butter, lemon, pepper, garlic, oil, salt, thyme, and mustard in your slow cooker. Switch the slow cooker on high and melt the butter.

2. Add the chicken; ensure to coat the chicken with the butter mixture.

3. Cook on low for 6 hours or on high for 4 hours. Add the cheese and let it sit for 15 minutes on low.

4. To serve, place the chicken over a bed of lettuce leaves.

Nutritional Value per Serving:

Calories: 280

Fat: 23.3g

Carbs: 4.1 g

Protein: 14g

Dinner

Kingly Kale Crispy Chips

Prep time: 4 minutes

Cook time: 12 minutes

Serves: 1

Ingredients

- 1-bunch large kale, rinsed, drained, and stemless
- 2-tbsp olive oil
- 1-tbsp salt

Directions:

1. Preheat your oven to 350°F.
2. Place the kale in a plastic bag. Pour the oil, and mix well by shaking the bag until coating thoroughly each leaf.
3. Spread the kale onto a baking sheet. Press the leaves flat to obtain an evenly crisped cook for each leaf.
4. Bake for 12 minutes until the edges turn brown while the rest of the kales remain dark green.
5. Sprinkle the salt over the baked kale and serve.

Nutritional Value per Serving:

Calories: 81

Fat: 7.6g

Carbs: 2.1 g

Protein: 1.9g

Day 21:

Breakfast

Healthy Breakfast Burritos

Prep time: 5 minutes

Cook time: 10 minutes

Serves: 4

Ingredients

- 8 eggs

- 1 tbsp milk

- 1 tbsp garlic, minced

- 1 red pepper, minced

- Half an onion, red if possible, minced

- 4 slices of bacon, cooked

- Salt

- Pepper

- 4 tortilla wraps (multi-grain or wholegrain)

- little cheese (optional)

Directions:

1. Take a medium sized saucepan and heat over a medium heat

2. Add the garlic and cook for a couple of minutes, until fragrant

3. Whisk the eggs with the milk and place to one side

4. Add the pepper and onion to the pan and allow to cook for a couple more minutes

5. Add the eggs to the pan and cook for 4 minutes

6. Once cooked, add a quarter of the egg mixture onto each tortilla wrap and add one piece of the bacon on top

7. You can add cheese if you want, although it isn't necessary

8. Wrap up and enjoy!

Nutritional Value per Serving:

Calories: 352

Carbs: 22g

Fat: 20g

Protein: 8 g

Lunch

Lentil Casserole

Prep time: 10 minutes

Cook time: 70 minutes

Serves: 8

Ingredients:

- ½ tsp. thyme
- 1 ½ cup green lentils, rinsed
- 1 lb. brown mushrooms, sliced
- 1 large onion, diced
- 1 tsp. garlic powder
- 12 oz. cream of mushroom soup
- 2 cup water, boiled
- 2 large carrots, diced
- 3 large stalks celery, diced
- 3 tbsp. extra virgin olive oil
- 4 oz. mozzarella cheese, shredded
- Sea salt & pepper to taste

Directions:

1. Start by preheating the oven to 375° Fahrenheit and put oil in a large dish for baking with cooking spray or oil of your preference.

2. Over medium heat, preheat a medium skillet with olive oil in it.

3. Add onion, celery, and carrots to the skillet and allow to cook for about five minutes, stirring throughout. Into the baking dish, empty into the skillet, then take the skillet back to the heat with more olive oil.

4. Kick the heat up to high and add the mushrooms to the skillet. Let them brown a little bit, then add them into the baking dish.

5. Return the skillet to the heat once more, dropping the heat down to low. Add oil, garlic powder, and thyme to the skillet, stir thoroughly, then add the lentils. Let that heat through for about two minutes, then add the water to the skillet.

6. While the water comes to a boil, use your spatula to light graze the bottom of the skillet to loosen the fond that has accumulated there.

7. Once boiling, add the soup to the pan and stir completely, adding more pepper and sea salt as is needed. Kill the heat and scrape the mixture into the baking dish. Thoroughly incorporate all ingredients in the dish and smooth it into one even layer.

8. Use foil to cover the dish and then bake for 30 minutes.

9. Remove the foil and return the dish to the oven for another 15 minutes.

10. Sprinkle cheese on top of the casserole, then return to the oven for up to five minutes or until the cheese is bubbly.

11. Let stand about 20 minutes to allow the dish to firm up, then serve hot!

Nutritional Value per Serving:

Calories: 267

Carbs: 35g

Fat: 9g

Protein: 15 g

Dinner

Cool Cucumber Sushi with Sriracha Sauce

Prep time: 20 minutes

Cook time: 0 minutes

Serves: 4

Ingredients:

For the Sushi:

- 2-pcs medium cucumbers

- ¼-pc avocado, thinly sliced

- 2-pcs small carrots, thinly sliced

- ½-pc red bell pepper, thinly sliced

- ½-pc yellow bell pepper, thinly sliced

For the Sriracha Sauce:

- 1/3-cup mayonnaise

- 1-tbsp sriracha

- 1-tsp soy sauce, gluten-free

Directions:

1. Slice one end of the cucumbers, and core them by using a small spoon to remove the seeds until completely hollow.

2. By using a butter knife, press the avocado slices into the center of each cucumber. Slide in the carrots and bell peppers until filling up completely each cucumber.

3. To make the dipping sauce, whisk to combine all the sauce ingredients in a bowl.

4. Slice the cucumber into 1"-thick round pieces, Serve with sauce on the side.

Nutritional Value per Serving:

Calories: 110

Fat: 10.1g

Protein: 1.9g

Carbs: 4.8 g

Conclusion

Now that you have learned about the process of intermittent fasting, it is time that you start practicing it too. Of late, this subject has gained a lot of attention, and people all over the world have received some amazing results. There are a lot of topics involved in intermittent fasting and if you learn them in-depth, you will realize the processes that go on behind the scenes. If you keep thinking about starting tomorrow, that tomorrow will never come. So, go ahead and start now. Even if it means abstaining from food for a few hours, do it. Then you can work your way up to twelve hours or more. Skip meals and maintain your diet. Do it regularly.

With time, you will realize that you have built the mindset that is required to follow balanced fasting. You will also become aware of the habits that you have inculcated when it comes to diet, and the moment you realize that you will be able to make the healthy shift necessary to maintain good health. Also, it is important that you ease into your fasts and not rush into it. Rushing will only make you impatient and disappointed. Once you fast consistently for about a month or more, you will see the results for yourself and your energy levels will drastically improve.

All the best !

Lightning Source UK Ltd.
Milton Keynes UK
UKHW022052200521
384096UK00003B/273